THE RETAIL REVOLUTION IN HEALTH CARE

THE RETAIL REVOLUTION IN HEALTH CARE

Myron D. Fottler and Donna M. Malvey

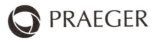 PRAEGER

AN IMPRINT OF ABC-CLIO, LLC
Santa Barbara, California • Denver, Colorado • Oxford, England

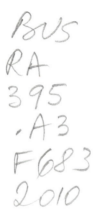

Copyright 2010 by Myron D. Fottler and Donna M. Malvey

All rights reserved. No part of this publication may be reproduced, stored in a retrieval system, or transmitted, in any form or by any means, electronic, mechanical, photocopying, recording, or otherwise, except for the inclusion of brief quotations in a review, without prior permission in writing from the publisher.

Library of Congress Cataloging-in-Publication Data

Fottler, Myron D.
   The retail revolution in health care / Myron D. Fottler and Donna M. Malvey.
      p. ; cm.
   Includes bibliographical references and index.
   ISBN 978–0–313–36623–9 (hard copy : alk. paper) — ISBN 978–0–313–36624–6 (ebook)
1. Health care reform—United States. I. Malvey, Donna M. II. Title.
[DNLM: 1. Delivery of Health Care—economics—United States. 2. Ambulatory Care Facilities—economics—United States. 3. Ambulatory Care Facilities—trends—United States. 4. Marketing of Health Services—methods—United States. 5. Patient Satisfaction—United States. W 84 AA1 F761r 2010]
RA395.A3F683   2010
362.1´0425—dc22   2009050896

ISBN: 978–0–313–36623–9
EISBN: 978–0–313–36624–6

14 13 12 11 10   1 2 3 4 5

This book is also available on the World Wide Web as an eBook.
Visit www.abc-clio.com for details.

Praeger
An Imprint of ABC-CLIO, LLC

ABC-CLIO, LLC
130 Cremona Drive, P.O. Box 1911
Santa Barbara, California 93116-1911

This book is printed on acid-free paper ∞

Manufactured in the United States of America

I would like to dedicate this book to my wife, Carol, for her patience during all the times I have been preoccupied with discussing, researching, and writing this book. As a result, I have not always been "in the moment." I also dedicate this book to my two dogs—Abby the Labby and Charley the Doodle. They helped to keep me focused on what is important in life, like good food, walks, playing with others, and sleeping. Finally, I would like to dedicate this book to a recent UCF master's program graduate, Megan McLendon, without whom this book would never have been completed. We wish her much success in her new career in health care administration.

—Myron Fottler

This book would not have been possible without the support and encouragement of lifelong friends who share my passion for improving our health care system. I would particularly like to thank Nancy and Rick Pounds, proprietors of Associates In Rehab (Lexington, Kentucky). During a visit to their clinic in 2005, they asked me why Walmart was opening in-store health clinics. At that time, few were even aware of what retailers were doing. Their simple question sparked my quest to discover why retailers were entering health care markets. In addition, I would like to recognize Elaine L. Cruz who provided essential research and editorial assistance in compiling our bibliography.

—Donna Malvey

Contents

Chapter 1

Introduction: Welcome to the Revolution

Rising health care costs, consumer discontent, and voter dissatisfaction have created fertile ground for radically changing the health care system. But which direction will change take us? Will it be toward the adoption of a national health plan that is government controlled? President Barack Obama's health reform plans emphasize more government control, including the possibility of a national health plan. Or is there another option emerging from the private sector? During the past decade the private sector has been quietly entering health care markets and innovating away from existing health care delivery systems and structures that do not work. In particular, large retailers have been experimenting with a variety of health service delivery models and products that promise affordable and convenient health care.

More than a decade ago Former Speaker of the House of Representatives Newt Gingrich predicted that health care was going to end up under the control of either the government or the marketplace. There would no longer be a middle ground; the existing health care system that combines both private and public structures and markets would disappear.

> One of the challenges I've made to doctors is, I said you're either going to go to Canada or to Wal-Mart. You can either go to a nationally controlled bureaucratic structure or you can go to the marketplace. But you are not going to stay in a guild status where you have all of the knowledge, you share none of it. (Gingrich, 1995)

The Speaker's predictions appear to be gaining ground in the twenty-first century, especially with respect to the retail giant, Walmart. Walmart, the largest retailer in the world, has entered health care markets in a manner commensurate with its size and purchasing power.

Among the innovations that Walmart has adopted are reduced prices for prescription drugs ($4 drugs), in-store primary care services (retail clinics), and (most recently) digital record systems for physician offices. Along the way, Walmart has teamed up with other industry giants, including Dell Computer, thereby making their impact in health care markets even more substantial. There clearly is some type of bandwagon effect occurring as more and more retailers join Walmart in the health care marketplace, including Target, CVS, and Walgreens. These retailers are bringing a new mentality to health care: efficiency, increased productivity, convenience, affordability, and transparency.

William Sage (2007) reminded us of Speaker Gingrich's perceptive remarks from 1995 in his recent article, "The Wal-Martization of Health Care." Sage assumed that going to Canada meant the United States would adopt a national health insurance, but going to Walmart meant shifting to a competitively run system to reform health care delivery. He detailed the emergence of a retail medical movement and concluded "Well, we have not gone to Canada. It is possible we are going to Wal-mart" (2007, p. 504).

RETAIL CLINICS

The new mind-set of retailers is evident in the emergence of the retail clinics, which offer a new model for primary care services that is based on service convenience and affordability. These clinics sell basic services to consumers at low prices and at convenient times and locations. These clinics are sponsored by large retailers, including pharmacy and grocery chains, and are located on their premises. These clinics are staffed by nurse practitioners, which are less expensive than primary care physicians. The market for basic primary care services seems to represent the largest untapped health care market. And retailers have carved out a niche for basic care that includes common illnesses such as colds, ear inflections, allergies, and preventive care such as immunizations.

Retail clinics emerged in 2000 with the opening of the first retail clinics in Minnesota. Since that time, over 1,000 clinics have opened in the United States and estimates indicated there may be as many as 6,000 of these clinics by 2011 (Scott, 2006). Their growth has spawned the Convenient Care Association, a Philadelphia-based organization founded in 2006 to represent retail clinics (Porter, 2008); publications such as the *Retail Clinician* that address issues associated with retail clinics; and national conferences and meetings such as the Retail Health Clinic Summit that is dedicated to best practices for retail health clinics. The retail clinic model continues to evolve to include *branding* through partnerships with hospitals and health systems, including prestigious institutions such as the Cleveland Clinic.

No Frills Health Care

Retail clinics also represent a concept that is new to health care: *no frills* health care that is offered at *bargain* prices. The care is provided by a physician substitute such as a nurse practitioner at a much lower cost to the consumer. The clinics are located within retail stores, pharmacies, and supermarkets. Patients spend little time waiting to be seen, and prescriptions are filled before they leave the premises. This is a walk-in business, with no appointments to schedule.

The concept of *no frills* health care appears to suit consumers' needs. Consumers appear to be willing to be treated by a less expensive provider such as a nurse practitioner in exchange for convenience and affordability (Mehrotra et al., 2008). Even in Massachusetts, known for its elite medical facilities, retail health clinics are thriving. Patients may see world class physicians for serious conditions, but if they get a bladder infection or sore throat on the weekend, the nurse practitioner down the street in a CVS drugstore will suffice for a simple health care problem (Kowalczyk, 2009).

Recent studies have affirmed that convenience is important to consumers, and they value the convenience that is offered by retail clinics. Most people are extremely busy today, balancing jobs and families. Multitasking is a way of life for most people, and consequently consumers look for convenience in most aspects of their life. Time has become a valuable commodity, and consumers look for ways to reduce waiting time such as using take-out or prepared foods or drive-by dry cleaning services.

As such, retail clinics are meeting needs for convenience that have not been previously satisfied in the existing health care system (Scott, 2006; Thygeson et al., 2008). Harris Interactive polling also reports high patient satisfaction with retail clinics (Harris

Interactive, 2008, May 21). And the Deloitte Center for Health Solutions reports that retail clinics are well received by patients. Furthermore, retail clinics have the potential to be *game changing* because of their affordability and convenience (Keckley, Underwood, & Gandhi, 2008).

The first major empirical study of retail clinics, funded by the Rand Corporation, reported that consumers also might prefer convenience over a particular provider relationship. Within a limited scope of services such as basic primary care services, the physician relationship may be less important to the consumer than convenience. The study also found that most of the retail clinic visits were for simple conditions and preventive care such as earaches, colds, and immunizations. As such, they probably do not merit the level of training of a physician. Finally, the study revealed that retail clinics actually appeared to be serving a patient population that may be underserved by primary care physicians. Given the shortage of primary care physicians, it is not surprising to learn that many who visit retail clinics may not have a primary care physician. Consequently, retail clinics could possibly function as a safety-net provider for patients who previously had no alternative for basic care other than the emergency department (Mehrotra et al., 2008).

Why are consumers accepting of health services delivered in a retail store setting? One possible explanation is past experience with self-care and home care. Over the years, consumers have gotten used to performing a variety of routine health care tests and treatments on their own, without physician authorization or supervision. Changes in reimbursement coupled with advances in technology have created an environment in which consumers not only have the ability, but often are required to provide health care services at home. Whether it is a home pregnancy test or over-the-counter remedies for acid reflux, consumers routinely purchase and use a variety of retail products instead of visiting a physician's office as they would have done previously.

In addition, many of the products that consumers use are sold in discount establishments. For example, early pregnancy testing products are now available in stores that sell goods for one dollar. Furthermore, during the 1980s hospitals began to discharge patients earlier because of reductions in reimbursement and to divert surgical procedures to outpatient facilities. Consequently, the patient or the patient's family was tasked with providing home care services after the surgery. Nowadays, patients themselves are expected to provide a variety of self-care services at home, ranging from self-injections to kidney dialysis, to changing catheters. Accordingly, patients have become accustomed to bypassing the physician's office and relying on themselves.

The concept of *no frills* service has been successful in a variety of other industries, too, where consumers appear willing to forgo certain high end amenities in exchange for lower prices and/or convenience. More than 30 years ago, U.S. consumers embraced self-serve gas stations in exchange for less expensive gas. More recent examples include the airline industry (Southwest Airlines) and investments (E*Trade). Southwest Airlines promoted steep price reductions in exchange for fewer amenities in the cabin and reserved seating. And E*Trade offered investors the opportunity to reduce charges for purchasing and trading stocks by eliminating the middleman, the stockbroker.

Health Information Technology

Retailers are advancing their move into health care markets with early adoption of health information technology. Unlike most hospitals and physician practices, retail clinics were early adopters of electronic medical records and computerized treatment protocols that sustain evidence-based medicine. Walmart is using its size and market power to sell an affordable digital health records system to U.S. physicians. Walmart has partnered with computer industry giant Dell, Inc., and software maker eClinicalWorks to produce an electronic health records package for physicians, which includes both installation and maintenance. The program will be offered through the company's Sam's Club discount-warehouse division and will undercut rival health information technology suppliers by as much as 50 percent (Lohr, 2009; Perrone, 2009).

Even though the government has promoted the adoption of electronic medical records for over a decade, these efforts have met with little success. Digitalized systems are costly to purchase, about $124,000 per single physician. In addition, the cost of installing and maintaining these systems is prohibitively high, especially for small physician practices.

Subsequently, despite the government's promotion, fewer than 20 percent of U.S. physicians currently use an electronic medical record. However, Walmart's entry into the market with an affordable health information technology product combined with the administration's targeted economic stimulus package incentives to encourage adoption of digitalized systems may just accomplish what the government set out to do more than a decade ago: improve the nation's health information technology. Not incidentally, Walmart used their in-store retail clinics to test the digital health records system that will be marketed to physician offices (Perrone, 2009; Lohr, 2009).

Innovation

When something does not work in the public sector, the government is reluctant to let go and usually continues to invest more resources, including money and people, in the hope of achieving success. There is little incentive for the government to "pull the plug" on programs because funding is always available through tax increases and deficit spending. The government has continued to try to fix the failing health care system for the past 40 years. Even though the public, politicians, and policy makers, as well as health care professionals, have predicted its collapse, the health care system continues to survive because the government has continued to invest in it (Brown, 2008). In fact, government spending for health care has increased to almost 50 percent and is expected to rise even more if there is an increase in government intervention (Lutz, 2008).

By contrast, when a concept or model does not work in the private sector, it is quickly rejected or revised if possible. Business cannot afford to continue to invest money and other resources in solutions that do not work or do not hold the promise of turnaround. Business cannot turn to the taxpayers for additional monies nor can it use deficit spending to fund its programs. Instead, business innovates to achieve increased inefficiencies.

Nowhere is there a better example of how business innovates to improve efficiencies than retail clinics. For example, Walmart continues to test and revise its existing retail clinic model. The company has adopted a telemedicine model at six retail clinics inside Walmart stores located in the Houston area. For this venture, Walmart partnered with a Houston-based retail clinic company, My Healthy Access, Inc., and NuPhysicia LLC, a commercial entity that was created in 2007 to implement telemedicine methodologies developed by the University of Texas Medical Branch at Galveston. This clinic uses doctors and paramedics instead of nurse practitioners. The telemedicine technology enables doctors to connect with clinic patients via video links installed in their offices or homes (Perrin, 2008).

The retail approach to health service delivery is very different from traditional medical offices where being patient is inherent in being one. Patients wait to get appointments, wait in offices for tests and treatments, and wait to find out how much it will cost them. Contrast this with a retail approach where the patient's needs come first. Retail clinics charge reasonable prices, which are usually advertised, do not require appointments, are open nights and weekends, have ample parking, and are in places where pre-scriptions can be filled. Their low cost and affordability have made the clinics a popular choice, especially for those without health insurance (Consumer Reports, 2009, April).

Retailers have introduced innovations to health care that tran-scend the conventional boundaries of the health care industry and ignore the restrictions of the institutional forces that work to ensure the status quo. Retailers consider patients to be consumers who have choices and deserve great service at a competitive price. If the service does not meet their expectations, retailers expect that consumers will go elsewhere (Crounse, 2008). The incentive for repeat business is what retailers bring to the table along with their persistence and ability to find ways to bring costs down.

Thus, while the government and politicians continue to devise excessively complicated and possibly unrealistic health reform plans, the private sector seems to be actually doing something to address key problems of access and cost. Thus far, retail clinics have addressed structural issues such as labor, overhead, and tech-nology in a way that has not previously been done in health care (Scott, 2006).

The movement of retailers into health care also appears to have spurred the growth of both employer-based or company clinics and also urgent care clinics. Company clinics were seen at the turn of the twentieth century, when large industries employed physi-cians to treat employees on site. Often there were few health care providers or facilities available to meet the needs of employees (Starr, 1982). Today large corporate employers are returning to the concept of the company clinic to reduce health care costs and ensure that their employees receive quality health care.

Examples of large companies that have adopted these clinics include North American Units of Toyota and Nissan, Harrah's Entertainment, Rosen Hotels, and Walt Disney Parks and Resorts. Toyota Motor, which revolutionized the auto industry, built an on-site medical center at its truck factory in San Antonio, Texas, at the cost $9 million in 2007. Despite the cost, the on-site facility is expected to save the company millions of dollars in the long run. Toyota's goals are to reduce health benefits expenditures, ensure a healthy workforce, and see increased productivity gains because workers will spend less time away from the plant for medical visits (Welch, 2008).

Urgent care clinics, often referred to as "doc in the box" facilities, which have been around for two decades, are also witnessing explosive growth. These clinics respond to consumer needs for extended hours and walk-in services for acute illnesses and injuries. The cost of their services are moderate compared with most physician office visits (approximately $120), and much less than an emergency room visit. Because these clinics provide for acute care, they are physician staffed (Consumer Reports, 2009). The Chicago-based Urgent Care Association of America, the largest trade group representing these clinics, estimates clinic numbers to be around 8,000 nationwide (Hendrick, 2008).

THE FUTURE

We clearly face two very different possible futures for health care. One possible future involves transforming health care by increasing government's role in it. In the 2008 election, voters expressed their discontent and dissatisfaction with the existing health care system. They overwhelmingly elected Democrats who support a national health plan that would expand access to health care and cover the uninsured. For the first time, the United States appears willing to adopt a more socialized approach to health care such as those offered in western European countries. In doing so, the United States would radically transform its existing health care system that is based on a complex evolution of public and private sector roles. It would complete, through health insurance, FDR's New Deal vision of social insurance as a fundamental American principle (Sage, 2007).

But whether this radical transformation occurs remains to be seen. If the economic crisis worsens or is extended for several years or if there is another terrorist event or natural disaster, priorities other than health care reform will likely occupy the government's attention.

A second possible future arises from what we call a "Retail Revolution in Health Care." We believe that transformative changes are being driven in large part by the private sector, in particular, big box retailers such as Walmart and Target, giant pharmacy chains like Walgreens and CVS, and entrepreneurs. These companies have redefined health care as a commodity to be bought and sold. They have tapped into consumer discontent and identified new health care markets and models of delivery that are more responsive to consumer needs and wants.

Retailers permit consumers to be in control so that they are able to use their spending power to effect significant alterations in the health care system. In the Retail Revolution, consumer preferences for convenience and affordability are taken seriously. Retailers are offering attractive options to respond to unmet consumer needs. Success will depend on consumers and choices that they make. In the Retail Revolution, the consumer is in charge—not the government and not insurance companies.

Because retail health care is much less expensive and access to care does not depend on having health insurance, consumers may naturally move in this direction. As more employers drop health insurance as a benefit and as layoffs continue, consumers will be looking for alternative means of obtaining health care. A recent survey of employers by Hewitt Associates, Inc., revealed that 19 percent of employers plan to stop offering health benefits over the next three to five years. This percentage is nearly five times as high as the 4 percent of employers who reported plans to drop health benefits in 2008 (Wojcik, 2009).

Mainstream news publications such as *U.S. News & World Report* inform us that *revolutionary* changes are already occurring in the delivery of health care services. Increasingly, patients bypass physicians to be treated by less expensive physician substitutes such as nurse practitioners (Gearon, 2005). The X Prize Foundation, which helped launch the first privately manned space flight in 2004, has partnered with the insurer WellPoint to offer a $10 million prize to anyone who can come up with a revolutionary idea to fix the health care system (Murphy, 2008). Yet, instances of revolutionary change are quite rare in health care.

There are only two documented examples of revolutionary or discontinuous change in health care. The first occurred in 1965 with the entry of the federal government into health care as a major purchaser through the Medicare and Medicaid acts. The second occurred in 1982–1983 when the federal government established a prospective payment system and introduced diagnosis related groups (DRGs). These interventions drastically revised the delivery of health care services because reimbursement and incentive structures shifted from cost-based to resource usage (Scott, Ruef, Mendel, & Caronna, 2000). But dramatic change does not guarantee positive outcomes. In the end, these revolutionary changes failed to fix the health care system and unwittingly contributed to ongoing problems and escalating health care costs.

Retail is a very powerful concept. The health care industry would do well to take note of what occurred in the banking industry in the late 1960s. The banking industry was conservative and not customer-centric. Banking hours were inconvenient for customers as banks were open weekdays, usually from 9 AM to 5 PM, when most customers were at work. Banks also charged fees for a variety of services including checking accounts. But the industry was upended when a few bankers began to conceptualize banking in retail terms; that is, money was a commodity to be bought and sold. This view led to the adoption of extended banking hours, which offered customers increased access, including late evenings and Saturdays. Drive-up windows were also adopted to ensure convenience for customers. Free checking reduced the cost of banking, and gifts such as toasters and television sets were offered as incentives to customers to open new accounts. As expected, banking customers embraced affordability and convenience.

Walmart and other retailers recognize that customers have needs and wants that are currently not being met by traditional health care providers. As such, these customers are fair game in the retail business, and the retailers are hotly pursuing them.

Will there be a revolution in health care? It appears so. The question is, who will lead the revolution and what will be its outcome? Will the government take control and create a nationally controlled bureaucratic structure that is similar to Western European nations? Will retailers reshape the health care industry much the same way that Toyota revolutionized the auto industry in the United States? Either way, the revolution is under way.

Who Should Read This Book and Why?

Health care is in crisis today. Costs are rising, quality is deteriorating, and access is limited. This book unveils and demystifies a *revolution* that is occurring in health care in the United States and beyond, and the changes it will bring. Retail health care represents real change and not more of the same. It seems to match the current "will" of the people at this moment in history. These changes can be expected to dramatically alter the health care landscape for all of us, especially key stakeholders ranging from patients to physicians, to hospitals and other providers, to insurers—even the federal government.

Yet few are aware of what is occurring in retail markets. As Table 1.1 illustrates, there are important rationales for reading this book for a variety of stakeholders. Key stakeholders, including consumers, health care professionals, politicians, and health policy makers have no comprehensive source of information on the retail health care phenomenon.

TABLE 1.1   Who Should Read This Book and Why

Key Stakeholder	Rationale for Reading this Book
Employers & Benefits Managers	Concern for containing costs while offering employees health care benefits, which ensure employees are healthy and productive and do not spend unneeded time away from work. Looking for the best health care products that are appropriately priced to enhance the employer's competitiveness rather than detract from it.
Health Insurers	Concern for keeping costs down so that they can pass these reductions on to employers and enhance their market share.
Health Care Providers (includes physician practices, hospitals, long-term care facilities)	Looking for ways to compete with retail clinics or enter into collaborative relationships.
Consumers/Patients	Looking for attractive options for health care that respond to their needs for affordability and convenience.
Educators	Looking for potential employers for graduates of their training programs in the health professions.
Politicians & Policy makers	Interested in cost containment and less costly options that can be easily implemented.

This book examines in depth the emergence and growth of retail health care, that is, the provision of primary health care services to consumers by various retail outlets such as Walmart, CVS, Publix Super Markets, Walgreens, etc. In addition, we examine partnerships among clinics and institutions, including hospitals and health insurers as well as the growth of these clinics globally. Retail clinics are growing exponentially across the United States and also emerging internationally. However, little information on them is available, especially in book form. Given current and projected shortages of primary care physicians and overcrowded emergency departments, retail clinics have the potential to fill a void. Health care is a political priority in the United States. Retail clinics most likely will play a key role as either an alternative to national health insurance or a component of health reform (Sage, 2007). These clinics enhance cost effectiveness, quality, and access, as well as respond to consumers' desire for convenience.

No previous book has examined the phenomenon of retail health care in part or comprehensively. This book presents a comprehensive overview of the retail health trend and its implications for consumers, employers, health care providers, health care companies, insurers, and health policy makers. We begin by identifying what is wrong with health care, the major "hassles" that consumers and providers experience. Next, we examine the phenomenon of retail health care from an entrepreneurial perspective, discussing the growth of retail care beyond traditional retail establishments, and possible performance indicators to assess health outcomes. We report on the differing perspectives of retail care from a variety of experts, including doctors, nurses, patients, and insurers. Finally, we address business realities both in the United States and around the world, including who supports and who opposes the growth of retail clinics and why. We will not only look at the present *state of the art*, but we will also take a futuristic view of the likely status of retail medicine in the future.

REFERENCES

Brown, D. L. (2008). The amazing noncollapsing United States health care. *New England Journal of Medicine, 358*(4), 325–327.

Consumer Reports. (2009, April). When you need care fast. *Consumer Reports on Health*, 6.

Crounse, B. (2008). *Healthcare goes retail: In-and-out checkups*. Retrieved April 5, 2009, from Microsoft Health Care Providers, Microsoft Health Care Providers Official Site: http://www.microsoft.com/

industry / healthcare / providers / businessvalue / housecalls / retail healthcare.mspx.

Gearon, C. J. (2005). Medicine's turf wars. *U. S. News & World Report, 138* (4), 57–60, 62, 64.

Gingrich, N. (1995). Newt's brave world. *Forbes*, 92.

Harris Interactive. (2008, May 21) *New WSJ.com/Harris Interactive Study Finds Satisfaction with Retail-Based Health Clinics Remains High.* Retrieved April 5, 2009, from Harris Interactive Official Site, Harris Interactive: http://www.harrisinteractive.com/news/allnewsby date.asp?newsid=1308.

Hendrick, B. (2008). *Urgent care centers seeing explosion in growth.* Retrieved March 17, 2009, from *The Atlanta Journal-Constitution*: http://www.ajc.com/search/content/business/stories/2008/06/ 27/boxdocs_0629.html.

Keckley, P., Underwood, H. R., & Gandhi, M. (2008). *Retail clinics: Facts, trends and implications, Deloitte Center for Health Solutions.* Retrieved April 5, 2009, from Deloitte Official Site: http:// www2.deloitte.com/assets/Dcom-UnitedStates/local%20Assets/ Documents/us_chs_RetailClinics_230708.pdf.

Kowalczyk, L. (2009). *Sick flocking to in-store clinics.* Retrieved April 5, 2009, from Boston Globe Official Site, boston.com: http://www .boston.com / news / health / articles / 2009 / 03 / 12 / sick_flocking _to_in_store_clinics/.

Lohr, S. (2009, March 11). Wal-Mart plans to market digital health records system. *The New York Times*, p. B1.

Lutz, S. (2008). Happy together: Consumer expectations for a public-private healthcare system. *Journal of Healthcare Management, 53,* 149–152.

Mehrotra, A., Wang, M. C., Lave, J. R., Adams, J. L., & McGlynn, E. A. (2008, September/October). Retail clinics, primary care physicians, and emergency departments: A comparison of patients' visits. *Health Affairs, 27*(5), 1272–1282.

Murphy, T. (2008). *WellPoint, X Prize launch $10M health care contest.* Retrieved April 5, 2009, from abcNews: http://www.azstarnet .com/sn/byauthor/262636.

Perrin, M. (2008). Retail health clinics re-open with new model. *Houston Business Journal.*

Perrone, M. (2009). *Wal-Mart to enter electronic medical records arena.* Retrieved April 5, 2009, from Yahoo Official Site, Yahoo News: http://news.yahoo.com/s/ap/20090311/ap_on_bi_ge/wal_mart _medical_records_2.

Porter, S. (2008). *Study examines role of retail health clinics: They may have role as complementary health care professionals.* Retrieved April 5, 2009, from American Academy of Family Physicians: http:// www.aafp.org/online/en/home/publications/news/news-now/ professional-issues/20080918randstudyretail.html.

Sage, W. M. (2007). The Wal-Martization of health care. *The Journal of Legal Medicine, 28*, 503–519.

Scott, M. (2006). Health care in the express lane: The emergence of retail clinics. *Report prepared for the California Healthcare Foundation.*

Scott, W. R., Ruef, M., Mendel, P. J., & Caronna, C. A. (2000). *Institutional Change and Healthcare Organizations.* Chicago, IL: The University of Chicago Press.

Starr, P. (1982). *The Social Transformation of American Medicine.* New York: Basic Books.

Thygeson, M., Van Vorst, K., Maciosek, M. V., & Solberg, L. (2008). Use and costs of care in retail clinics versus traditional care sites. *Health Affairs, 27*(5), 1283–1292.

Welch, D. (2008). *Health-Care Reform, Corporate-Style.* Retrieved April 5, 2009, from Business Week Official Site, Business Week: http:// www.businessweek.com/magazine/content/08_32/b4095000246 100.htm.

Wojcik, J. (2009). *19% of employers plan to drop health benefits.* Retrieved April 5, 2009, from Business Insurance: http://www.business insurance.com/cgi-bin/news.pl?newsid=15654.

Chapter 2

What Is Wrong with Health Care Today?

The U.S. health care system reportedly is a growth industry. It is also considered to be America's largest service industry. U.S. government economists predict that public and private health care spending will reach $2.5 trillion in 2009 or 17.6 percent share of the gross domestic product (GDP) (Reuters, 2009). More than 14 million people are employed in this segment of the economy, and these numbers are expected to increase even during the economic downturn (Bureau of Labor Statistics, 2008–2009).

On the other hand, those who work in and study the U.S. health care system have consistently regarded it to be on the verge of economic collapse. For more than four decades, the system has been in financial crisis and survived because of increases in government spending for health care. The federal government funds public health insurance programs such as Medicare and Medicaid, hospital building programs as well as research, education, and training programs of health professionals (Brown, 2008).

For all intents and purposes, it would seem that the U.S. health care system has been participating in a long-term government *bailout* program. Unlike recent government bailouts for banks, insurance companies, and automobile manufacturers, which have involved significant amounts of money in the short term, the health care bailout has been incremental and has occurred over 40 years. The government now pays nearly half of the bill for all health care that is consumed in the United States and is expected to soon become the majority payer (Lutz, 2008). If a national health plan is implemented, the government will control American's largest service industry, health care.

However, an increase in government spending over the years does not appear to have fixed the health care system. Instead, the system has come to depend on state and federal funds for survival. It seems that during the course of every election, politicians and consumers complain about the health care system, especially its skyrocketing costs, and demand change. While Congress has enacted major policy initiatives intended to control health care costs, all have failed to achieve suggested objectives. Provider initiatives for cost containment have failed, too.

What is left to do? Attempt more of the same? Or is it time to implement something radically different; let the government assume complete control over health care? However, there is little if any evidence that indicates the government has the solutions to fix the health care system. Perhaps it is time to look at alternative solutions emerging in the retail sector such as retail health clinics.

What is wrong with health care today? Regardless of whom you ask the question, whether it is a patient, physician, or politician, the answers are invariably the same: *The health care system is broken. Health care costs too much. It is not meeting my needs and wants.* Patients will complain about time spent waiting to see a doctor or getting an appointment. They will also complain about the actual visit with the doctor because it is too brief and there is no time to ask questions. Patients also grumble about the paperwork, lack of transparency, and escalating out-of-pocket costs. If patients are seeking specialty medical care for chronic illnesses such as diabetes and arthritis, their complaints will increase because of additional appointments with doctors and diagnostic facilities for testing. If people lose jobs, they will complain more because of the loss of their health insurance. If they are forced to find insurance in the private markets, it will be expensive and cover fewer services.

Doctors protest, too. Similar to patients, doctors also object to the increase in paperwork and administrative detail. Overhead costs are rising and reimbursement rates are failing to keep pace with rising costs so that doctors must see greater numbers of patients to maintain income levels. Consequently, the time that doctors have to spend with patients is diminishing as well, making it more difficult for doctors to maintain their relationships with patients. Doctors are particularly worried about the patient relationship because it has been the cornerstone of their authority in medicine (Starr, 1982). They are also worried about the time and effort it takes both them and their staff to address the needs of aging baby boomers who present with multiple chronic illnesses (Tang & Lee, 2009).

Other health professionals criticize the health care system, too, because they are forced to do more with less. Nurses have higher patient loads, pharmacists fill more prescriptions, and physical therapists treat patients with multiple problems. Hospitals complain about the impact of reimbursement cuts on their budgets and their ability to furnish care for the uninsured. As the impact of the economic downturn spreads, hospitals are cutting needed services.

For example, Nevada has been particularly hard hit by the recession. Many of its residents have lost their health insurance because of rising unemployment. Nevada's public hospitals, which have been the safety net for the poor and uninsured, have had to close programs because of the financial crisis. University Medical Center discontinued its outpatient cancer clinic, meaning that its patients will no longer be able to obtain chemotherapy and other cancer treatments at the facility. Because many patients are without health insurance or on Medicaid, they have few alternatives. The seriousness of this cutback drew the attention of CBS *60 Minutes*. The nation watched as patients with cancer talked about their prognosis without chemotherapy and other treatments (CBS *60 Minutes*, 2009).

Academics and others who study health care do not give it high marks, either. The Commonwealth Fund Commission (2006) reported that the U.S. health system fell far short of achievable benchmarks for health outcomes, quality, access, efficiency, and equity. In a National Scorecard on U.S. Health System Performance, the United States received a score of 66 (out of a possible 100 points), which is one-third below benchmark levels of performance. Despite such dismal results, the U.S. health care system continues to function. Year after year, the government continues to invest in it without seeing any improvement in health outcomes. Why has the federal government continued to sustain a health care system that performs so poorly?

THE U.S. HEALTH CARE SYSTEM HAS NOT BEEN ALLOWED TO FAIL AND IT SHOWS

Because the U.S. health care system is sustained by government spending, it never has been allowed to fail. This is one of the potential problems identified with the government bailing out an industry. The government continues to prop up failing systems and in doing so tolerates inefficiencies that the private sector would not (Scandlen, 2005). In fact, the private sector uses failure as a guide to eliminate inefficiencies and refocus its objectives. Thus, unlike the public sector, the private sector learns what contributes to success and what causes failure.

Nowhere is this distinction more evident than in an evaluation of system outcomes for the U.S. health care system: cost, access, and quality. Every one of the major problems in U.S. health care is associated with these system outcomes. Yet attempts to reshape the health care system have focused primarily on controlling costs, thereby ignoring important aspects of access and quality and the impact of cost reductions on those outcomes.

As Table 2.1 illustrates, over the years, neither government nor private sector initiatives have succeeded in controlling rising health care costs or in achieving improvements in system delivery. In 1964, the government intervened in health care by way of legislation that created two public health insurance programs: Medicare, which increased access to health care for the elderly, and Medicaid, which furnished health services for the very poor. Health care spending dramatically increased as Americans began accessing health care through these programs.

In 1974 the federal government introduced the Health Planning and Resource Development Act, which created Certificates of Need (CON) that give local and state agencies authority to review and approve or disapprove hospital capital expenditures. The goal was to reduce duplication among facilities and encourage hospitals to share expensive equipment and technologies. But even though there was some cost savings, the cost of medical care continued to increase faster than the consumer price index through the 1980s (Shortell, Morrison, & Friedman, 1990, pp. 4–5).

Prior to October 1983, when prospective payment legislation was enacted, most hospitals were reimbursed on a cost basis (i.e., for the full costs of patient care). A prospective payment system replaced cost basis with predetermined fixed payment levels for 468 diagnostic related groupings (DRGs). Hospitals that could provide care within payment limits could keep the savings. Those that could not were forced to absorb the loss. This marked the first time that there was a national systematic incentive for hospitals to behave efficiently (Shortell, Morrison, & Friedman, 1990, pp. 4–5).

During the 1980s, entrepreneurs launched ventures aimed at achieving more efficient services and enhancing the quality and

TABLE 2.1   Summary of Private and Public Sector Initiatives

Timeframe	Initiative	Sector	Outcomes
1960s	Medicare/Medicaid	Public	Medicare costs have skyrocketed to the point where it faces an uncertain future. Medicaid has cut reimbursements to providers so that many physicians and facilities will not accept Medicaid payment for services.
1980s	Prospective Payment System (PPS) and Diagnostic Related Groupings (DRGs)	Public	Did not effectively control costs. PPS rewarded intensity of care and resource usage so that hospitals and physicians focused less on primary care services and more on highly reimbursed services such as cardiac surgery. Providers shifted many operations to outpatient environment to avoid DRGs.
1980s	Entrepreneurial ventures. Physicians launch ventures such as ambulatory clinics, sometimes with hospitals as partners. Hospitals legally and functionally reorganize to engage in business ventures, many of which are non–health care. Entrepreneurs open health care businesses such as mobile CT scans.	Private	Entrepreneurs failed to achieve success in many ventures because they did not understand the business of health care. Similarly, hospital attempts at non–health care ventures also had many failures. Hospitals found that the cost of joint venturing with physicians was prohibitive. Entrepreneurs failed because of obsessive growth and expansion and single-minded focus on marketing rather than delivery of service (Herzlinger, 1989).

1990s	Clinton Health Plan Initiative	Public	Failed to gather support for implementation.
1990s	Insurers grow in power as they implement tightly controlled managed care, with physician gatekeepers. Hospitals engaged in vertical integration: mergers, acquisitions, and consolidation. Hospitals purchased physician practices in order to secure market segments.	Private	Managed care held costs down for a brief period, but caved in to a backlash from physicians and patients over access to care issues. Hospitals failed to control costs through vertical integration, growth, and accumulation strategies. Merger attempts were unsuccessful or resulted in hospital cultures that clashed. Hospitals learned that purchasing physician practices reduced physician productivity as well as incentives to enhance revenues.
2000s	Retail health clinics: Retailers quietly enter the health care market by sponsoring retail health clinics in their stores.	Private	By 2009, there were almost 1,000 retail clinics across the United States. Patients report high rates of satisfaction with them. The clinics offer basic health care at low cost.
2009	Democratic administration calls for national health plan.	Public	Details and outcomes are unknown at this time.
2009	Providers offer new ways to deliver service, especially electronically, including e-medicine, telephone consultations, the medical home concept, and grouped patient visits. Retailers continue to experiment with new service delivery methods such as telemedicine.	Private	Details and outcomes of health care reform are unknown at this time.

accessibility of care (Herzlinger, 1989). Physicians also became entrepreneurs by establishing ambulatory surgical centers and diagnostic facilities. In some cases, they entered into joint ventures with hospitals to operate these facilities. In other cases, they competed directly with hospitals for patients. At the end of the decade, few entrepreneurs succeeded in revitalizing the health care system. Entrepreneurial efforts of the 1980s failed to put patient needs and wants first. Instead, entrepreneurs focused on growth, marketing, and restructuring sources of capital to generate high returns (Herzlinger, 1989, p. 98).

In the 1990s, the Clinton Health Plan failed to achieve consumer or industry support and also did not gain Congressional approval (Sage, 2007). Private sector insurers responded with initiatives to control costs through managed care. In the 1990s managed care organizations used nurse practitioners and physicians as gatekeepers to restrict patients from unnecessarily using health services, particularly specialty care, and redirect patients to less expensive primary care services. There was a backlash from both consumers and physicians about such gatekeeping activities. Physicians especially objected to second-guessing of their clinical decisions as well as reductions in their payments (Robinson & Ginsburg, 2009).

In the 1990s, hospitals consolidated operations and developed systems and networks that were aimed at cost reductions rather than satisfying consumers. Many hospitals acquired physician practices as a means of gaining control over the most expensive system input. Physicians were put on the payroll, but hospitals quickly learned that physician productivity declines when physicians do not have a financial stake in their practice. Subsequently, hospitals divested themselves of their physician practices.

It was not until 2000, when retailers entered the picture that we began to see priority consideration given to what consumers want in terms of service delivery, especially convenience and affordability. Unlike doctors and hospitals, whose tasks and payments are predetermined by insurers, retailers are free to package and price their services to respond to consumer needs and wants. As a result, beginning in 2000 we saw the emergence of retail health clinics in large discount stores, pharmacy chains, and supermarkets (Goodman, 2009).

In 2007 at the World Health Care Congress, which was held in Washington, D.C., Walmart's president and CEO, Lee Scott, gave the closing keynote speech. In his remarks, he shared information about plans to open health care clinics in Walmart stores and for

Walmart to partner with providers around the country. The retail movement that he spoke about is very focused on using technology to ensure a patient experience that reflects convenience, affordability, quality, and safety (Goodman, 2007).

Why Have So Many Attempts Failed?

One of the likely explanations for continued failure of both public and private sector initiatives is an erroneous assumption that there is a "one size fits all" solution for reforming a $2.4 trillion health care system (Dentzer, 2008, p. 1217). It has been argued that the health care system puts the value of powerful interests before the value of patients. Powerful interests include physicians, hospitals, drug companies, and insurers, which are well-organized and well-funded. They use their influence in the development of strategies for reimbursement and regulation that ensure their financial benefit. Powerful interest groups also oppose innovations that do not support their status in the health care system. Even when the government funds demonstration projects that have the promise of innovation, the projects tend to be designed by and favor the powerful stakeholders in the health care system. Thus, patients are essentially left out of the process (Lee & Lansky, 2008).

Also, most of the reform initiatives have focused on revising the insurance models and financing mechanisms and not on fixing actual service delivery problems such as convenience. Even though the majority of Americans (more than 80 percent) have health insurance, public sector initiatives have mainly focused on efforts to revise insurance methodologies (Sage, 2007; Dentzer, 2008, p. 1216). During the past 50 years, Democrats have persisted in working to obtain insurance coverage for all Americans, and with the election of a Democrat president in 2008, they are unlikely to change their direction (Iglehart, 2009). Thus, we can expect government to continue focusing on insurance models and financing systems to reform health care. There is little if any evidence to suggest that the government will initiate efforts to fix delivery system problems such as lack of convenience for the consumer.

TEN CORE PROBLEMS

In order to fix the health care system, it is essential to identify the main problems that afflict it. Below is a list of ten core problems that we believe contribute to the poor performance and reputation of the U.S. health care system.

Problem #1: The U.S. Health Care System Is Bipolar

The U.S. health care system is bipolar in terms of its organizational structure and also in terms of the politics that influence it. This means that the health care system has two spheres of influence: public and private. In terms of structure, the system is a constellation of both sectors. The U.S. health care system contains both private and public hospitals. Hospitals can be owned and operated by private companies, local communities, and state and federal governments. Approximately 25 percent of the nation's community hospitals are independent. Furthermore, facilities dedicated to public health are limited. Most are on the periphery of the health care system despite the potential increase in public health disasters such as bioterror events.

The U.S. health care system is also criticized as being a nonsystem because of the fragmentation that arises from combining both public and private sector components (Brown, 2008). This is especially true in terms of sources of funding, which can be private, public, state, local, and federal sources. Fragmentation is also reflected in terms of physician organization and practice. Some physicians are hospital based such as pathologists and anesthesiologists. However, most physicians are in private practice. More than half of all doctors work in small practices of three or fewer doctors. There is also diversity within specialized sectors of the health care industry. For example, biotech and medical device manufacturers and suppliers are also represented by thousands of small firms (Herzlinger, 2006, p. 61).

The health care system is also bipolar from a political perspective. Health care reform has reflected political divisions, with liberals calling for increased access to health care, usually through universal health insurance. Meanwhile conservatives have voiced opposition to further government intervention and called for free market solutions. Even though both liberals and conservatives agree that health care costs must be contained, their approaches to doing so have been subordinated to their main concerns of access and government intervention. Because the U.S. health system contains both public and private components, it is a system that is based on *accommodating* both sets of interests. Even though both public and private sector interests are concerned with cost containment, only the private sector simultaneously focuses on ways to increase profitability as well.

For years the business community has chosen to align itself with conservative solutions and opposed a national health insurance mostly because of its opposition to increased government regulation. It successfully opposed the Clinton administration's efforts to reform health care in the early 1990s because of excessive regulation (Sage, 2007). However, in 2008 the business community was less predictable. The rising cost of employer health insurance seemed to have persuaded many business owners that it was preferable to embrace a national health plan. A national plan would guarantee their employees health care, which would be paid for in large part by the government instead of the business owner. Furthermore, a national plan would shift the responsibility for health care from business to the government.

Problem #2: No One Is in Charge, Accountable, or Responsible

No one person or entity is in charge, responsible, or accountable for the health care system's performance. Even if the government assumes complete control over health care, authority and decision making will likely be diffused through a massive bureaucratic structure. Once again, no one will really be in charge or held accountable for system outcomes. Does anyone want to be responsible for health care? No one in the public sector is stepping up to the plate.

In the public sector, it is common to find responsibility for a particular area shifted to specially created boards. For example, the Federal Reserve Board was created to assume responsibility for monetary policy. The Federal Aviation Administration was established to oversee the airline industry. More recently, the call is to create a separate entity to assume responsibility for health care. President Obama's former nominee for secretary of Health and Human Services (HHS), Senator Tom Daschle, proposed establishing a separate board to assume responsibility for health care.

In his recent book, *Critical: What We Can Do about the Health Care Crisis* (2008), Senator Daschle proposed creating a Federal Health Board, composed of political appointees who would be assigned responsibility for health policy decision making. Daschle writes, "I suspect that most members of Congress would be glad to be rid of their responsibility for controversial health policy decisions" (p. 199). The idea that Congress would abdicate their responsibility for health care seems particularly self-serving, especially in view of

2008 campaign promises. However, even though Daschle withdrew his nomination as secretary, the plan for a separate health board has been incorporated in the various health reform proposals.

But it is not only the public sector that does not want to be held accountable for health care. It is also private sector insurers. In the past, insurers have opposed health reform proposals, including the Clinton plan of the 1990s. But in December 2008, the health insurance lobby, America's Health Insurance Plans (AHIP), put forth their own proposal for health reform. The AHIP asserts that their plan reflects the result of several years of work and a multicity "listening tour" conducted by health insurers. This proposal is the third from AHIP since Democrats took control of Congress in the 2006 election.

The most recent proposal builds on the existing system, but adds a requirement for individuals to buy insurance. The industry plan suggests a 30 percent reduction in projected growth of national health expenditures, but provides few details on achieving this goal. Congress would be responsible for setting a target for sustainable national health spending and also for establishing an advisory group that would actually make health policy proposals to achieve the target (Armstrong, 2008). The proposed advisory group would relieve Congress of responsibility for making health policy and in this regard is similar to Daschle's plan for a Federal Health Board. Thus, while it seems that while everyone calls for change in the health care system, few are willing to step up to the plate and be held accountable for the outcomes of any change.

Problem #3: The Patient Has Not Been Empowered

In the past decade, efforts have been made to empower patients to exercise more control over resource usage. However, thus far it appears that patient empowerment is limited. When patients are sick, they want to get better. They are not concerned with efficiency and minimizing use of resources. Furthermore, how are consumers expected to learn about appropriate use of system resources when they do not have complete information? Because there is little transparency in the health care system, consumers are mostly in the dark when it comes to much of the medical decision making.

The market for medical care does not perform like other markets. Providers normally do not disclose their prices prior to treatment (Herrick, 2008). When a consumer visits a doctor's office, there is no menu board listing the prices, and the consumer has no way of knowing what type of financial relationship the physician has with the insurer, suppliers, and drug manufacturers. Insurance companies create networks of providers, negotiate discounts for services, and offer physicians performance incentives. Meanwhile, physicians write orders for patients to obtain services. Choices that patients make about using health system resources (i.e., whether to see a particular physician or use a hospital service) often are taken out of the patient's control altogether and are assumed by insurers or plan administrators (Herrick, 2008).

Increasingly, patients also are held responsible for their health outcomes. For example, women are advised to eat healthier and exercise to prevent their getting breast cancer. However, there is no definitive evidence that adequately supports such advice. We do not know why some women get breast cancer and others do not. There are many women who eat healthy foods, exercise, and still get breast cancer.

Furthermore, it is assumed that if consumers become educated about their disease and treatment options, they will make better decisions about using health care resources. Yet much of the medical information that is available to the consumer has not been authenticated, especially from Web sites. There are growing problems of unreliability with information for consumers and also the potential for information and medical advice to be tainted by conflict of interests. Even top tier medical journals have learned that they published medical studies without being informed that these studies were funded by drug companies and others with vested interests in study outcomes (Brownlee, 2007).

Problem #4: The U.S. Health Care System Is Perpetually in Crisis

Health care is perceived to be perpetually in crisis, especially financial crisis. More recently, the crisis has added the uninsured as a new dimension, but the financials continue to dominate. Consequently, health reform efforts over time have been directed toward the controlling costs. However, none of the efforts to control costs have ever been effective. Health care costs continue to climb, and health care spending increases each and every year (Starr, 1982, p. 381; Fuchs, 2009; Brown, 2008; Oberlander, 2009; Christensen, Bohmer, & Kenagy, 2000).

Making decisions while in crisis mode is not the optimal way to function. In crisis situations, one's judgment is often impaired by looming catastrophic events. Decisions are made quickly and with a view toward short-term solutions and outcomes. When the roof is falling in, no one stops to do strategic planning. Instead, stopgap measures are adopted to avoid further disaster. For over 40 years, attempts have been made to fix the health care system with short-term stopgap measures. What has occurred is analogous to what takes place in a trauma or intensive care unit of a hospital. The patient, which in this case is the health care system, is kept alive and stabilized.

However, longer-term issues such as maintaining that steady state or preventing reoccurrence of the problem are not adequately addressed, if at all. Thus, while government spending has managed to keep the health care system from collapsing, it has not fixed systemic problems (Brown, 2008). The health care system has a pulse, but is still very sick.

Problem #5: The U.S. Health Care System Tolerates Inefficiencies

Health care appears to be distinct from other industries because it tolerates inefficiencies. Innovative firms in other industries can go directly to the consumer with innovations, but in health care it is hard to get to the consumer directly. As such, innovations are not influenced by consumers (Pauly, 2008). Special interests in the industry exert undue influence and opposition in adopting innovations. These powerful groups advocate for the status quo because they will not benefit from change. In doing so, these groups ensure that the health care system tolerates inefficiencies, especially in service delivery.

The health care industry has failed to adopt changes, especially low-cost disruptive innovations, which are believed to foster revolutionary change and improve the delivery of health care services. According to innovative disruption theory, these innovations disrupt the status quo by enabling less-skilled workers to perform the work of expensive highly trained specialists in more convenient and less expensive settings (Christensen, Bohmer, & Kenagy, 2000).

Such disruptions have succeeded in radically altering other industries. For example, photocopiers now permit office workers to perform printing inexpensively and to do things that previously only professional printers could do at much higher cost. An example of disruptive innovation in health care is using software that incorporates standardized practices to permit non-physician clinicians to provide preventive, chronic, and basic medical care (Andrews, 2005).

However, the retail movement in health care represents the emergence of disruptive innovation in the health care system (Keckley, Underwood, & Gandhi, 2008). Large retailers are using their size and influence to change the way care is delivered. From affordable prescription drugs to retail health clinics, retailers are taking health care directly to the consumer. In doing so, they are bypassing providers and insurers. They are packaging and pricing health care services to suit the consumers' needs and wants.

Problem #6: Health Care in the United States Is Unaffordable

Americans are worried about rising health care costs and how they will pay for health care. The annual Health Security Index survey, commissioned by Catholic Healthcare West, measures perceptions of consumers' confidence about health care. The 2009 Security Index revealed more Americans are worried about health care costs (69 percent) than losing their jobs (39 percent). Furthermore, even the affluent are increasingly concerned about affordability of health care (Health Security Index, 2009). But a lack of confidence about health care is not only measured by perceptions. It is also reflected in the quantitative measurements that indicate that health care costs are out of control.

In 2007, the United States spent $2.4 trillion on health care, roughly 17 percent of its GDP or $7,900 per person (National Coalition on Health Care, 2009). Health care spending is expected to grow to $4 trillion or 20 percent of the GDP within a decade (Commonwealth Fund Commission on High Performance Health System, 2006).

The United States spends more on health care than any other country. Even though the United States has fewer physicians, nurses, and hospital beds per capita than other industrialized countries, it still manages to outspend them. Furthermore, it outspends them despite the fact that Americans reportedly go to the doctor less, are admitted to hospitals less frequently, and have shorter lengths of stay when admitted in comparison to residents of other industrialized countries (Collins, Schoen et al., 2007, p. 18).

The United States spends twice as much as Japan on health care, but there is no evidence that our health care is twice as good (Mahar, 2006). The U.S. often ranks with or below third world countries in certain disease categories and infant mortality. In addition, Americans spend twice as much on out-of-pocket expenses as do residents of other industrialized countries (Collins et al., 2007, p. 18). If there is no evidence that increased spending on health care makes Americans healthier, why does the United States continue to spend huge sums of money on a health care system that does not achieve basic system goals?

Researchers have studied such questions for years and produced statistical data that offer some detail but no definitive answers. For example, from research we know that hospital and physician and clinical services represent the largest components of health care spending, 31 percent and 21 percent, respectively. Prescription drugs account for 10 percent of spending, which is a 40 percent increase during the past 40 years (Centers for Medicare and Medicaid Services, 2008). But we do not know which factors specifically contribute to cost increases. Are costs rising because of high administrative expenses, escalating payments to hospitals and physicians or the practice of defensive medicine? Again, there is no definitive answer.

There has been extensive examination of factors such as demographics (the aging of the population), administrative costs, medical practice, and technology. Some research has demonstrated that technology accounted for an estimated half to two-thirds of spending growth (Ginsburg, 2008). Unlike other industries, in which technology leads to cost reductions, health care technology advances seem to contribute to cost increases. For example, the CT scan, which was advancement over the X-ray, costs more. The MRI, which superseded the CT scan, costs more, too. And there have been charges of misusing and overusing the technology. In many cases, the simple less expensive X-ray is sufficient for diagnosis, but the more expensive technologies are used because of higher rates of reimbursement (Mahar, 2006, p. 178; Brownlee, 2007).

Both the private and public sectors have attempted unsuccessfully to control spending and reduce costs. Public sector initiatives to restrain costs have consistently focused on cost controls and payment reforms, that is, revising reimbursement methods. Yet payment reform is not system reform. Payment reform is narrowly focused and does not contribute to improvements in health service delivery. On its own, payment reform is more likely to realize unintended consequences that ultimately undermine its goals of cost containment and impede service delivery. For example, in the 1980s, the government attempted to restrain costs by shifting from cost-based reimbursement to a prospective system that was based on resource usage. The change in reimbursement systems failed to deter rising costs.

Some have suggested that the prospective payment methodology precipitated the move of physicians from primary care to specialty care because specialty care meant more resource usage and subsequently higher rates of reimbursement. This was the opposite of what was intended when the prospective payment system was implemented. The new system was supposed to incentivize hospitals and physicians to use fewer resources, but it soon became obvious that the incentives supported higher reimbursements for specialty care (Kahn, 2009). And today we face shortages of primary care doctors because the reimbursement methods initiated under the prospective payment system continue to reward specialty care.

The government's efforts to contain costs are often wiped out because they occur simultaneously with efforts to expand program benefits. Expansion of benefits serves to increase program use, which increases health care spending. For example, the privatized drug benefit for Medicare recipients resulted in a record 18.7 percent increase in Medicare costs (Kuttner, 2008). The rationale for expanding benefits at the same time the government is trying to reduce costs was obviously political.

Some would argue that it is the private sector which precipitates medical inflation. The private sector's emphasis on commercialization and profit maximizing behaviors are said to distort costs and resource allocation (Kuttner, 2008). However, health care has been openly operating like a business since the 1970s. Even nonprofits, including hospitals, pursue profitability to remain competitive with their for-profit counterparts in the industry. Furthermore, physician practices are typically for-profit enterprises. However, the trend toward commercialization of health resources has been recognized. In large part this is due to incentives in the system, most of which are determined by public policy initiatives, especially payment reforms (Starr, 1982; Mahar, 2006).

Managed care was once perceived to have the potential to rationalize the health care system, eliminate efficiencies, and reduce costs. But its aggressive cost controls ultimately failed to bring about major change in the health care system. Once managed care loosened its strict controls, physicians and hospitals eventually reverted to their earlier behaviors. They are once more competing aggressively, especially for profitable specialty and ancillary services that yield higher payment rates and contract terms. Providers tend to invest in technology that is well compensated. The outcomes of this type of competition have been a buildup of capacity for increasingly expensive services and technology as well as escalating costs (Lesser and Ginsburg, 2003).

Both public and private insurers have attempted to reduce costs through utilization controls by increasing deductibles and levying co-pays and co-insurance fees to deter patients from unnecessary visits to the doctor and diagnostic tests. However, if a patient has a condition that requires the care of a specialist, sending that patient to a primary care doctor who may have little experience in the area does not make economic sense. The primary care doctor is likely to try a variety of treatments, requiring multiple visits, and ultimately refer the patient to a specialist. On the other hand, the specialist may be able to resolve the problem in one visit.

Take the case of Linda. In the 1990s Linda was a college student, still covered under her parent's health insurance. She presented to the primary care physician with a rash, sore throat, and fever. On the first visit, she was diagnosed with the flu. A week later she returned because she had not gotten any better. This time, the doctor focused on the fact that Linda was a college student and might have mononucleosis. Tests did not confirm this diagnosis. Linda returned again and again because she continued to get worse. The primary care doctors continued to do tests that yielded little information and insist that this was a particularly bad outbreak of the flu with a prolonged recovery period. Eventually, Linda's mother took her to the Emergency Department, where Linda was admitted to the hospital. Linda did not have the flu. She had a severe reaction to a medicine that had been prescribed for her acne, minocycline. Her kidneys and neurological systems were affected and recovery lasted over one year. The cost of not referring Linda for specialty care was considerable to the health plan and to Linda. Today, most private health plans permit patients to self-refer to specialists because it makes economic sense.

Problem #7: Access to Health Care Is Limited by Multiple Factors

Access to medical care is a challenge in the United States because it involves overlapping problems. First, there is the issue of access to health insurance. Many in the United States cannot get access to health care because they lack health insurance. A visit to the doctor's office requires an insurance card or some type of guarantee of payment. Second, there is the problem of access that involves availability of clinics, hospitals, doctors, nurses, and others who provide care. Just having health insurance will not guarantee access to health care, especially if there are shortages of facilities and health care workers.

There are already in the United States severe shortages of a wide range of health care workers, including primary care doctors and nurses. If the uninsured, estimated to be 47 million persons, were to be given health insurance, where would they go for care and treatment? They would have to use existing facilities, which means that they would show up either at already overcrowded doctors' offices or overcrowded emergency departments. And for the uninsured who reside in rural areas, they will be particularly challenged because rural areas already face scarce resources in terms of facilities and providers.

The United States is the only industrialized nation whose citizens are not guaranteed access to health care. The Health Research Institute at PricewaterhouseCoopers identified its top list of concerns for health executives and policy makers in 2009. Among the top concerns were the uninsured and the rapid growth of the underinsured. Specifically, the number of underinsured was growing faster than the number of uninsured. Since 2003, the number of underinsured has increased 60 percent. It has been estimated that as many as 47 million people in the United States are without health insurance and another 25 million who have health insurance are actually underinsured and could not meet expenses for a catastrophic illness such as cancer. These people have health plans with high deductibles and co-pays, which means that they have to pay more out of pocket for health services (PricewaterhouseCoopers' Health Research Institute, 2008).

Currently, health insurance is offered by most employers for full-time employees. But even the employed are increasingly without insurance because their employers can no longer afford to offer it. Public insurance programs exist for the very poor (Medicaid) and for people 65 years of age and older (Medicare and supplemental programs associated with Medicare coverage). There are also private insurance markets that offer health coverage, but these plans are usually quite expensive, have high deductibles, and have limitations on preexisting conditions.

Expanding access to health care will mean an increase in spending to cover the care of both the uninsured, at least 47 million, and the underinsured, at least 16 million. Furthermore, simply giving every American health insurance will not guarantee them access to health care. Additional facilities and additional health professionals will also be needed to provide treatment and care. However, while access to medical care is an incredibly difficult problem, especially for the uninsured, service delivery solutions have access advantages over insurance solutions (Sage, 2007, p. 515).

Problem #8: High Cost Does Not Necessarily Equal High Quality

Not all costs can be measured directly. Some costs occur in terms of loss of trust in the health care system by patients and also in terms of declining patient satisfaction. This is where issues of quality enter the equation (Kohn, Corrigan, & Donaldson, 2000). The United States may be outspending other countries, but it has not produced the healthiest population. The idea that high cost translates to high quality has generally been accepted in the United States (Davis & Cooper, 2003). Yet efforts to reduce costs and make the health care system efficient may be changing that translation, especially with insurers looking to negotiate steep discounts with providers. Still, one wonders if delivering high quality at low cost is merely a "wishful thinking mantra" (Pauly, 2008, p. 1352)?

For example, the government has increased health care spending during the past four decades, but the added financial support has yielded few quality improvements. Meanwhile, retailers have used health technologies such as electronic health records and standardized protocols to support quality improvements and evidence-based medicine.

There are emerging discussions that American health care actually may be doing harm while also doing good. Many patients appear to be overtreated or improperly treated for their conditions because much of the care that patients receive is not evidence-based (Brownlee, 2007; Mahar, 2006). "Evidence-based" means that the care and treatment prescribed are based on some evidence that the treatment will help the patient get better. When patients do not improve, they often may end up seeking help from another provider or attempting to obtain relief using over-the-counter remedies. Worse still, the patient may postpone seeking any type of care at all.

Studies have also shown that prescribed treatments will vary according to region of residence. For example, whether you have surgery or chemical treatment for prostrate cancer will depend on what the doctors in the community routinely do rather than evidence that shows a particular treatment is more effective for your case. Even though doctors routinely test for levels of prostate-specific antigen (PSA) to detect prostate cancer, there is no evidence that using the test improves survival (Carey, 2006; Andriole et al., 2009).

Patient safety emerged as a priority issue during the past decade. Approximately 98,000 were reported to die from medical errors annually, making it the fourth leading cause of death in the United States (Kohn, Corrigan, & Donaldson, 2000). Yet ensuring patient safety is a voluntary matter for most hospitals and facilities. Some oversight is provided by accrediting organizations and state licensing organizations. Although patient safety has attracted much media attention and subsequently been influential in publicizing the systemic problems, neither public nor private insurers underwrite the cost of patient safety initiatives and programs. Subsequently, a hospital will be reimbursed for resources used in performing a particular procedure such as removing an appendix.

However, none of the reimbursement includes funds dedicated to patient safety; that is, to ensure that the patient does not acquire a hospital-based infection during his hospital stay. The federal government has established a zero-tolerance policy for preventable hospital-acquired complications. As of October 1, 2008, the Centers for Medicare and Medicaid will no longer reimburse hospitals for the care of specific conditions if they are acquired as a direct result of hospitalization (HealthGrades, 2009).

In 2001, 18-month-old Josie King died from medical errors at the prestigious teaching hospital Johns Hopkins. To its credit, the hospital admitted responsibility and has committed to fostering a culture of patient safety. But the hospital's efforts were purely voluntary (King, 2002). Medication errors, both inside and outside of the hospital, can inconvenience, injure, and kill patients. Actor Dennis Quaid made the headlines in 2007 when his newborn twins were given an accidental overdose of a blood thinning drug, Heparin. The twins were given an adult dosage, which was 1,000 times the amount that they should have received. The actor subsequently sued the hospital (ABC News, 2007). Large pharmacy retailers also have been sued for prescription errors, some of which have been serious and resulted in death. Patients are also being harmed by acquiring infections while in the hospital, and some of these infections are potentially lethal such as MRSA.

Donald Berwick MD is co-founder and chief executive officer of the Institute for Healthcare Improvement (IHI), which is dedicated to improving quality and achieving effective care. Although IHI has realized some genuine progress in terms of saving lives, reducing medication errors, and shortening clinic wait times, Berwick believes that the U.S. health care system remains stalled and needs revolutionary change to bring about improvements in quality of care (Mahar, 2006, p. 181).

Regardless of what happens to the patient, payments are made to doctors and others who provide care. Because payment for service is independent of the outcome or results, treatments and tests are often prescribed without consideration of their effectiveness. Furthermore, unproven treatment regimens and overpriced drugs are often shown to be no better than what they replaced (Brownlee, 2007; Mahar, 2006).

For example, Patient A visits the family doctor for a routine exam. The doctor identifies that the patient's blood pressure is somewhat elevated and prescribes an expensive drug to reduce it. The patient develops some side effects from the medicine, so the physician either changes the drug or prescribes additional drugs to combat the side effects. The patient is then required to schedule follow-up visits to monitor the drug usage. Meanwhile, Patient B's visit to the physician is a completely different experience. The doctor recommends that the patient first start with lifestyle changes of diet and exercise to reduce blood pressure and suggests adding drug therapy only if the lifestyle changes fail to bring about improvement.

During the past 40 years, the U.S. health care system has become the most expensive in the world. Yet it is deficient in many respects, including patient safety and quality measures. In the public sector, one could conclude that a high price tag for health care does not necessarily translate to high quality health care. Despite government subsidies, there are cost increases. And cost increases are not commensurate with improvements in quality. However, the private sector is another matter altogether. Retailers are aiming to capture certain health care markets by offering quality care at affordable prices.

Problem #9: Consumers Are Not Driving the U.S. Health Care System

There is no standard definition for consumer-driven health care; however, consumer-driven health care has been conceptualized in terms of insurance models and financing (Scandlen, 2005). As a result, most consider it to mean a health benefit plan that is designed to give consumers more control over their health spending. Usually it involves a high deductible insurance plan with a personal account that funds payments for health care. The Health Savings Account (HSA) is a recent example. The primary notion underlying consumer-driven health care is that if the consumer writes the check, the consumer has some control of his spending for health care services. Meanwhile experts in consumer-driven health care, such as Regina Herzlinger, argue that a true consumer-driven approach must involve providers and consumers in more than payment decisions. Consumers must be involved in decisions about care delivery, including making it better and less expensive (Herzlinger, 2002, p. 45).

The underlying assumption of giving the consumer some *direct* control over his health spending decisions is that the consumer will make choices based on efficient use of resources. However, this assumption seems to imply that consumers are otherwise *out of control* when it comes to making decisions about how they spend their health care dollars. Even though consumer-driven health care is intended to make consumers directly responsible and accountable for their health spending decisions, it raises questions about how consumers make health care decisions. For example, do we really expect the parents of a sick child to make choices based on efficiency? If we did, we would also expect to find children with terminal illness in hospice care. But we do not.

When someone becomes ill, he usually wants to do everything possible to get better. The U.S. health care system is committed to going *all the way* to save patients. This is in stark contrast with western European health care systems that practice rationing of health care. For example, in England those over 70 years of age would not expect to receive organ transplants because they are in competition with much younger recipients. Or heart surgery might be deferred because of age and health conditions. Meanwhile, in the United States, we expend resources with a view toward saving lives, not conserving resources.

Consumer-driven health care might make perfect sense to economists and others who study health care with assumptions of rationality. But it makes less sense in the context of illness, especially serious illness. Consumers might defer seeking care because they cannot afford it. In doing so, they become much sicker. Conversely, some consumers will disregard economic considerations altogether and spend for survival.

Consumer-driven health care is also problematic because it does not suggest how we may empower the poor whose spending decisions are restricted by limited resources. Nor does it provide guidance for those who are very sick and also very poor. How do we empower these consumers and put them in charge of health spending?

When consumers take control in other industries, such as retailing, banking, computers, or automobiles, they do so by applying pressure. The pressure is that they will go elsewhere if their needs and wants are not met. The outcomes are usually increased productivity and reduced prices. Choices are expanded and quality is improved (Herzlinger, 2002, p. 45). But in health care, consumers have few opportunities to use pressure tactics because they typically do not pay for their care directly.

As recently as 1960, U.S. consumers paid directly for 49 percent of all health spending. That amount gradually eroded as both public and private third party payers gained control over health care spending. In 2002, U.S. consumers paid only 14 percent directly; third party payers, both government and private insurers, were responsible for 86 percent of spending. As payment for third parties has grown, the health care system has become more expensive and less responsive to consumer needs and wants. Patients essentially became disconnected from a direct role in the health care system. Payers and other intermediaries perform as middlemen and control patient financial responsibility for their health care (Scandlen, 2005; Herrick, 2008).

Problem #10: The U.S. Health Care System Has Lost Sight of Its Customer

Just who is the customer in health care? In the 1990s, the health care customer was conceptualized as a *fluid* term, which includes anyone who receives a product or service such as patients, physicians, suppliers, payers, and even co-workers (Eisenberg, 1997, p. 25). This fluid definition complicates matters because health care organizations must develop strategies that meet and satisfy oftentimes competing needs of multiple customers. In doing so, they lose sight of who the real customer is—the patient. Even though the health care industry has focused on customer service and meeting consumer needs, the incentives and the customer are very different.

For example, in the hospital, the customer (patient) is not paying for the service. The primary customer for the hospital is the doctor who admits the patient. The secondary customer is the insurer who reimburses the hospital for services used by the patient. The patient's choice of a hospital is restricted to one that is acceptable for payment by the insurer and also one where the doctor has admitting privileges. The hospital ensures that the doctor is satisfied with the surgical suite, the equipment, the personnel, especially the nursing staff that will provide around the clock care for the patient, and anything else that the doctor needs. The hospital works to ensure that insurers get all documentation and paperwork necessary to process the reimbursement.

But what about the patient? The patient will likely be required to show up hours in advance of a hospital procedure and wait. The hospital will secure any copayments up front and require the patient to sign a statement stipulating responsibility for additional payments.

Even though statistical and perceptual evidence affirm that the U.S. health care system is in need of repair, they do not measure the discontent and dissatisfaction in the system, especially among consumers of health services. Survey questions often do not address what is at the heart of consumer concerns, especially convenience. Consumers wait everywhere for health care. They wait for appointments; they wait in the crowded doctor's office; they wait in overcrowded emergency rooms; they wait in line for prescriptions. Given today's hectic life style and multitasking, consumers are increasingly unwilling to waste time waiting. Because of the Internet and cellular communications, consumers are used to getting what they want any time and immediately. Why should health care be any different?

THE FUTURE

The President's Plan

President Obama believes that the health care crisis is tied to the economic crisis. We cannot fix one without fixing the other. However, elected officials have been trying to reform health care for decades and without much success. Costs have continued to escalate, consumer needs go unmet, and there is little innovation. We did not get where we are today without the help of politicians and their decision making. The president has indicated that he would like to expand access to health care to include the uninsured. This is a compassionate goal, one which is supported by most in the United States.

However, implementing this goal is problematic. Not only would it increase the federal budget, at a time when the budget is seriously challenged by bailouts, but it also potentially would create chaos in the health care system because (1) it does not reduce costs and (2) giving someone insurance does not mean that you are providing them access to health care services. To have access to health care, there must be health care facilities nearby and health professionals employed in those facilities to provide care and treatment.

The president's health reform proposal would enable those with employer-sponsored insurance to retain it if they want to. Large employers would be required to offer workers coverage or contribute a certain percentage of their payroll to support a new public plan. A health insurance exchange would be created through which people without insurance could select coverage through either private coverage or the new public plan at rates similar to those offered through large employers. Cost reductions are expected to be achieved by combating anticompetitive actions in drug and insurance companies, supporting disease prevention and health promotion efforts, and expediting adoption of health information technology (Iglehart, 2009).

Although the president's plan lacks specific details on key features, including sources of financing, it basically puts private insurance plans in direct competition with a public insurance plan. The Commonwealth Fund Commission on a High Performance Health System described this type of mixed approach as the most pragmatic because it builds on the best features of the existing system. It allows those people who currently have good health insurance to maintain it. The responsibility for paying for health care is shared with individuals, employers, and the government (Collins & Kriss, 2008).

Moving quickly was viewed as essential to current health reform efforts by President Obama and the secretary of HHS. He does not want to repeat the health reform failure of the Clinton administration that waited too long to get started. President Bill Clinton's health reform legislation did not emerge until the fall of his first year in office, 1993. Many felt that Clinton was distracted by foreign policy and other issues that diminished momentum for health reform (Wayne, 2008; Daschle, 2008). However, President Obama faces far more potential for distraction than President Clinton, including two wars and an economic recession that is reputed to be the worst in United States history since the Great Depression.

Obtaining public input regarding how to improve the health care system is also important. Obama's transition team has solicited the public's opinions on health care in a nationwide campaign. Community meetings and something called "house parties" were held in late December 2008 to gather information on health care concerns and experiences. Such efforts appear consistent with Obama's campaign promise to maintain transparency in the process of health reform and give the American people a direct say in health reform (Kaiser Daily Health Policy Report, 2008). However, the actual legislation developed in the House and Senate in fall 2009 is very much "top down" with an expanded role for the federal government and its various panels.

But what will the great *American Shout Out* really accomplish? Can a grassroots health reform approach fix the health care system? Health reform has been a top-down approach, where Democrats in Congress and the administration make the decisions. Is a bottom-up approach, which allows the consumer's voice to be heard, possible? Will special interest groups' needs and wants take precedence over the consumer once again? Thus far, no one really has been listening to consumers and their complaints about convenience and affordability. No one, that is, except for retailers.

The Retail Movement

Paradigm shifts may come from outside a particular industry because people within an industry can be too close to the problem to recognize potential solutions (Barker, 1993). In the health care industry, leaders from university medical centers and academic health institutions that led a generation ago, are still in charge. In the United States the history of health reform has been almost exclusively focused on efforts by government, insurers, and employers to control costs and not on improving how people get medical care (Sage, 2007). These entities have prevented consumers from exercising control within the industry (Herzlinger, 2002).

Instead of looking to any of these entities to fix the health care system, we might be better off looking at private sector initiatives and even outside the United States to other countries such as India, which has been successful in reducing costs for expensive cardiac surgeries (Dentzer, 2008). Within the U.S. private sector, retailers have identified large untapped consumer markets such as basic care. In addition, they have recognized that consumers value convenience and affordability, both of which are not being addressed within the existing health care delivery system.

A key feature of large retailers is they constantly reinvent their business models, performing ongoing assessments and reassessments of the "fit" between the services being offered and the desires of the buying public. Large retailers are always looking for ways to serve their customers better, and they recognize that profitability is reflected in their commitment to continuous improvement in service and convenience. Retailers have only one customer, the consumer of health services. And retailers are focused on serving that customer.

Conclusions

What is wrong with health care today? What is wrong with health care today is what was wrong with health care yesterday. All of the money spent on health care services originates from the consumer's pocket, but consumers have little control or authority over the system. Whether the payer is the government, insurance company, or an employer—every penny spent on health care comes from the consumer in the form of taxes, premiums, or earned compensation (Scandlen, 2005). Furthermore, the government and private insurers pay for care regardless of whether the care helps the patient to get better (Brownlee, 2007).

Health care reform initiatives have focused on controlling health care costs. But costs are a symptom of what is wrong with the U.S. health care system, and proposed solutions to rein in costs are likely doomed to fail much as they have done in the past. We have a dysfunctional, inefficient, and ineffective *delivery* system. Consumers do not get the care they need and want when they need it. And providers, both physicians and hospitals, are bottlenecked with red tape, regulations, and administrative bureaucracies.

Consumers of health care services have been *powerless* to change the health care system, depending on politicians and policy makers to make things right. And those who have benefited by this system, either directly or indirectly, have been reluctant to change it. Special interest groups have guaranteed the status quo in health care and advocate only for change that serves their particular *special* interest. It appears that radical or revolutionary change will be necessary to divest the health care system of the stranglehold of powerful institutional forces that are sustained by the status quo.

The U.S. health care system is not based on logic or rationality. It has evolved on the basis of political accommodation (Starr, 1982). Whether it has been politicians or special interest groups, decisions about the U.S. health care system have been made based on who gets what and who is more powerful, not the needs and wants of the consumer. But the cost of "accommodation" has taken its toll on both the U.S. economy and consumers. Business can no longer afford the skyrocketing cost of health insurance and remain competitive globally. The government cannot afford to keep pace with rising costs in the face of an unprecedented economic downturn. More important, the consumer is discontented not just with cost increases but with the inconvenience and treatments that often seem more like medical guesswork than science (Brownlee, 2007; Carey, 2006). Consumer discontent and dissatisfaction have intensified to the point where consumers are speaking with one voice. They want change in the U.S. health care system.

In the 2008 election, health care remained a top priority for most voters even when the economy and homeland security issues competed for top positions on their agenda. Voters in the United States indicated that they want the government to do something to fix the health care system even if it involved radical change such as a nationalized health insurance. However, health care is complex, and so many efforts engineered to reform the system have failed. Assuming that all the complexities and problems can be solved by giving the government control is unfounded. For decades the government has attempted to control costs without success. Why should we expect that giving the government more control over health care would not result in similar failure?

Can the Health Care System Be Fixed?

If past is prologue, we would expect the government to be the change agent and lead the way in transforming the health care system. But every public policy initiative thus far has failed to reform the health care system and has caused numerous unanticipated consequences. And every provider initiative has also failed to achieve reform objectives. What has been done thus far has *not* been truly customer focused. Consumer needs and wants have *not* been a priority.

What is needed are customer-focused initiatives, such as those promoted by retailers. Retailers know who the customer is and focus on improving service delivery. They measure the success of their efforts by satisfying the customer. Retailers focus on continuous service improvement to enhance customer satisfaction, whereas government programs tend to become ossified.

Beginning in 2000 with the first retail health clinics, retailers have been revising the boundaries and organizational structure of health care service delivery. They have done so by taking basic medical care out of the doctor's office. This is an example of transformative change. Consumers no longer have to go to a physician's office for primary care services. They can be treated for basic health care needs while shopping at a retail store, pharmacy, or even supermarket. And it does not end with basic health services. Walmart has begun to experiment with telemedicine business models that allow consumers access to a variety of physician services that can include specialty care.

In addition, it appears as if physicians are beginning to embrace such innovations as e-medicine and looking to treat patients' basic medical care needs electronically using the Internet and email. The patient can email or telephone a physician about a basic health care need to see if an office visit is required. SwifMD.com is an example of a Web-based company that offers such consultations with physicians for nominal charges such as $75 per physician consultation or reduced prices if the consumer obtains a membership subscription service.

In a landmark study of the nature and extent of changes in medical care delivery systems, Scott and colleagues (2000, p. 1) observed that change does not come easily to the health care system. However, when it does, profound changes can occur quite rapidly. But who will lead this change: the government or retailers?

REFERENCES

ABC News (2007, November 21). *Medical mistakes not uncommon in U.S.* *ABC News* Television Broadcast.

Andrews, M. (2005, February 1). *Gone in 60 seconds: An innovative chain called MinuteClinic is trying to reinvent the way you get treated for routine ailments.* Retrieved November 4, 2005, from CNN Money.com Official Site, Fortune Small Business: http://money.cnn.com/magazines/fsb/fsb_archive/2005/02/01/8250649/index.htm.

Andriole, G. L., et al. (2009). Mortality results from a randomized prostate-cancer screening trial. *New England Journal of Medicine, 360*(13), 1310–1319.

Armstrong, D. (2008, December 3). *Insurers offer own proposal for health care overhaul.* Retrieved April 14, 2009, from The Commonwealth Fund Official Site: http://www.commonwealthfund.org/content/newsletters/washington-health-policy-in-review/2008/dec/washington-health-policy-week-in-review—december-8–2008/insurers-offer-own-proposal-for-health-care-overhaul.aspx.

Barker, J. (1993). *Paradigms: The business of discovering the future.* New York: HarperBusiness.

Brown, D. L. (2008). The amazing noncollapsing U.S. health care. *New England Journal of Medicine, 358*(4), 325–327.

Brownlee, S. (2007). *Overtreated: Why too much medicine is making us sicker and poorer.* New York: Bloomsbury.

Bureau of Labor Statistics. (2008). *Career guide to industries, 2008–2009 health care.* Retrieved April 10, 2009, from United States Department of Labor, Bureau of Labor Statistics: http://www.bls.gov/oco/cg/cgs035.htm.

Carey, J. (2006). *Medical guesswork: From heart surgery to prostate care, the health industry knows little about which common treatments really work.* Retrieved April 15, 2009, from BusinessWeek Official Site: http://www.businessweek.com/magazine/content/06_22/b3986001.htm.

CBS *60 Minutes.* (April 5, 2009). *The Recession's impact: Closing the clinic— 60 Minutes: Bad economy leaves cancer patients without health insurance in dire straits.* Retrieved April 6, 2009, from CBS News Official Site: http://www.cbsnews.com/stories/2009/04/03/60minutes/main4917055.shtml.

Centers for Medicare and Medical Services. (2008). *National Health expenditures by type of service and source of funds, CY 1960–2006.* Retrieved April 7, 2009, from Centers for Medicare and Medical Services: http://www.cms.hhs.gov/nationalhealthexpenddata/downloads/quickref.pdf.

Christensen, C. M., Bohmer, R., & Kenagy, J. (2000, September 1). Will disruptive innovations cure health care? *Harvard Business Review,* Reprint R00501, 1–9.

Collins, S. R., & Kriss, J. L. (2008). The public's views on health care reform in the 2008 presidential election. *The Commonwealth Fund, 29.*

Collins, S. R., Schoen, C., Davis, K., Gauthier, A. K., & Schoenbaum, S. C. (2007). A roadmap to health insurance for all: Principles for reform. *The Commonwealth Fund, 73.*

The Commonwealth Fund Commission on a High Performance Health System. (2006, September 20). Why not the best? Results from a national scorecard on U.S. health system performance. *The Commonwealth Fund, 34.*

Daschle , T. (2008). *Critical: What we can do about the health-care crises*. (J. M. Lambrew & S. S. Greenberger, Narrators). New York: Macmillan.

Davis, K., & Cooper, B. S. (2003). American health care: Why so costly? *The Commonwealth Fund, 654*, 1–33.

Dentzer, S. (2008, September/October). Innovations: "Medical Home" Or Medical Motel 6? *Health Affairs, 27(5)*, 1216–1217.

Eisenberg, B. (1997). Customer service in healthcare: A new era. *Hospital & Health Services Administration, 42*(1), 17–31.

Fox, M. (2009, April 9). *Obama sets up formal office for healthcare reform*. Retrieved April 10, 2009, from Reuters Official Site, Reuters: http://www.reuters.com/article/politicsnews/idustre53801320090409.

Fuchs, V. R. (2009). Health care reform—Why so much talk and so little action? *New England Journal of Medicine, 360*(3), 208–209.

Ginsburg , P. B. (2008, October). *High and rising health care costs: Demystifying U.S. health care spending*. (Vol. The Synthesis Project, Issue 16). Princeton, NJ: Robert Wood Johnson Foundation.

Goodman, J. (May 2, 2007). *If Wal-Mart did healthcare . . . .* Retrieved April 7, 2009, from Microsoft Corporation, Worldwide Health for the Microsoft Corporation: http://blogs.msdn.com/healthblog/archive/2007/05/02/if-wal-mart-did-healthcare.aspx.

Goodman, J. (January 6, 2009). *FYI: Entrepreneurs go where doctors can't and third-party payers won't*. Retrieved April 10, 2009, from John Goodman Blog Official Site, John Goodman's Health Policy Blog: http://www.john-goodman-blog.com/entrepreneurs-go/.

HealthGrades. (2009, April). *HealthGrades releases sixth annual patient safety study results*. Retrieved April 14, 2009, from HealthGrades Official Site: http://www.healthgrades.com/media/dms/pdf/patient safetyinamericanhospitalsstudy2009.pdf.

Health Security Index. (2009). *Health security in America*. Retrieved April 10, 2009, from Catholic Healthcare West, Health Security Index: http://www.chwhealth.org/who_we_are/advocacy/stgss044099.

Herrick, D. (2006, January 1). *Demand growing for corporate practice of medicine*. Retrieved December 31, 2005, from The Heartland Institute: http://www.heartland.org/publications/health%20 care/article/18269/demand_growing_for_corporate_practice_of _medicine.html.

Herrick, D. M. (2008, December). *Health care entrepreneurs: The changing nature of providers, policy report no. 318*. Retrieved April 10, 2009, from the National Center for Policy Analysis Official Site: http://www.ncpa.org/pdfs/st318.pdf.

Herzlinger, R. E. (1989, March/April). The failed revolution in health care —The role of management. *Harvard Business Review, 67*(2), 95–103.

Herzlinger, R. E. (2002, July). Let's put consumers in charge of health care. *Harvard Business Review, 80*(7), 44–55.

Herzlinger, R. E. (2006, May). Why innovation in health care is so hard. *Harvard Business Review, 84*(5), 58–66.

Iglehart, J. K. (2009). Visions for change in U.S. health care—The players and possibilities. *New England Journal of Medicine, 260*(3), 205–207.

Kahn, C. N., III (2009). *Payment reform alone will not transform health care delivery.* Retrieved April 8, 2009, from Health Affairs Official Site, Health Affairs: http://content.healthaffairs.org/cgi/gca?allch= &SEARCHID=1&AUTHOR1=kahn&FULLTEXT=payment+reform + alone + will + not + transform + health + care + delivery & FIRST INDEX=0&hits=10&RESULTFORMAT=&gca=healthaff%3B28% 2F2%2Fw216.

Kaiser Daily Health Policy Report. (2008). *President-elect Obama's transition team solicits U.S. residents' opinions on health care in nationwide campaign.* Retrieved December 8, 2008, from Kaisernetwork.org: http://www.kaisernetwork.org/daily_reports/health2008dr.cfm? dr_id=55959.

Keckley, P., Underwood, H. R., & Gandhi, M. (2008). *Retail clinics: Facts, trends and implications: Deloitte Center for Health Solutions.* Retrieved April 5, 2009, from Deloitte Official Site: http://www.deloitte.com/ dtt/article/0,1002,sid%253d127087%2526cid%253d217872,00.html.

King, S. (2002). *What happened—Sorrel King's speech to the IHI Conference, 2002.* Retrieved April 10, 2009, from Josie King Foundation: http:// www.josieking.org.

Kohn , L. T., Corrigan, J. M., & Donaldson, M. S., Eds. (2000). *To err is human: Building a safer health system.* Authoring organization is the Committee on Quality of Health Care in America, Institute of Medicine. Washington, DC: National Academy Press.

Kuttner, R. (2008). Market-based failure—A second opinion on U.S. health care costs. *New England Journal of Medicine, 358*(6), 549–551.

Lee , P. V., & Lansky, D. (2008, September/October). Making space for disruption: Putting Patients at the center of health care. *Health Affairs, 27*(5), 1345–1348.

Lesser, C. S., & Ginsburg, P. B. (2003). Health care cost and access problems intensify: Initial findings from HSC's recent site visits. *Issue Brief of The Center for Studying Health System Change, 63*, 1–4.

Lutz, S. (2008). Happy together: Consumer expectations for a public-private healthcare system. *Journal of Healthcare Management, 53*, 149–152.

Mahar, M. (2006). *Money driven medicine.* New York: Harper Collins Publishers.

The National Coalition on Health Care. (2009). Health insurance cost: Facts on the cost of health insurance and health care. Retrieved April 15, 2009, from National Coalition on Healthcare Official Site: http://www.nchc.org/facts/cost.shtml.

Oberlander, J. (2009). Great expectations—The Obama administration and health care reform. *New England Journal of Medicine, 360*(4), 321–323.

Pauly, M. V. (2008, September/October). "We aren't quite as good, but we sure are cheap": Prospects for disruptive innovation in medical care and insurance markets. *Health Affairs, 27*(5), 1349–1352.

PricewaterhouseCoopers' Health Research Institute. (2008). *Top nine health industry issues in 2009: Outside forces will disrupt the industry.* Retrieved April 10, 2009, from PricewaterhouseCoopers' Health Research Institute Official Site: http://www.pwc.com/extweb/pwcpublications.nsf/docid/dcf3340a60807a328525751b00197e8c.

Robinson, J. C., & Ginsburg, P. B. (2009). Consumer-driven health care: Promise and performance. *Health Affairs, 28*(2), w272–w281.

Sage, W. M. (2007). The Wal-Martization of health care. *The Journal of Legal Medicine, 28*, 503–519.

Scandlen , G. (2005). Consumer-driven health care: Just a tweak or a revolution? *Health Affairs, 24*(6), 1554–1558.

Scott, W. R., Ruef, M., Mendel, P. J., & Caronna, C. A. (2000). *Institutional change and healthcare organizations.* Chicago, IL : The University of Chicago Press.

Shortell, S. M., Morrison, E. M., & Friedman, B. (1990). *Strategic choices for America's hospitals: Managing change in turbulent times.* San Francisco: Jossey-Bass Inc. Publisher.

Starr, P. (1982). *The social transformation of American medicine.* New York: Basic Books.

Tang, P. C., & Lee, T. H. (2009). *Your doctor's office or the Internet? Two paths to personal health records.* Retrieved April 1, 2009, from www.nejm.org, New England Journal of Medicine: http://content.nejm.org/cgi/content/full/360/13/1276.

Wayne, A. (2008). *He wrote the book on health care.* Retrieved December 8, 2008, from The Commonwealth Fund Official Site: http://www.commonwealthfund.org/content/newsletters/washington-health-policy-in-review/2008/dec/washington-health-policy-week-in-review—december-8–2008/he-wrote-the-book-on-health-care.aspx.

Chapter 3

The Top Ten Consumer Health Care Hassles

Americans experience a large number of specific hassles as they attempt to access health services for themselves and their families. Ten specific hassles are outlined in Table 3.1 in terms of their key characteristics and impacts on access, quality, and cost of health services. These hassles are very relevant to the subject of our book because they illustrate the kinds of health care challenges experienced by most Americans, which are in the process of being addressed by retail medicine. A major challenge in this book is to determine to what degree retail medicine might alleviate these hassles.

Recently, Harris Interactive surveyed a random sample of 1,004 U.S. adults on behalf of the Commonwealth Fund to determine their perspectives and experiences on the organization of the nation's health care system (How, Shih, Lau, & Schoen, 2008). Eight of ten respondents agreed that the health care system needs either fundamental change or complete rebuilding. The respondents' health care experiences underscore the need to ensure timely access, better coordination, and a better flow of information among doctors and patients. There is also a need to simplify health insurance administration. Finally, there was broad agreement that wider use of health information systems and greater care coordination could improve patient care by enhancing quality and access while containing costs.

Some of the specifics of the survey indicated the following (How et al., 2008):

TABLE 3.1   Top Ten Consumer Hassles

Problem/Hassle	Key Characteristics of Problem/Hassle	Impact on Access, Cost, and Quality		
		Access	Cost	Quality
1. Problems in getting appointments	• Do not take your insurance • Shortage of providers • Providers out of insurer's network • Overbooking of provider's schedule to minimize the impact of "no-shows"	X		
2. Long waits for services	Patients show up for appointments only to find that they must spend additional time in waiting areas • to see a physician, • for a diagnostic procedure • to pick up a prescription	X		X
3. Patients spend little time with physicians	• Paperwork and documentation decrease the time that physicians can spend with patients • Physicians are high cost providers and their time is specified by insurers		X	X
4. Administrative paperwork	• Documentation required for insurers, government agencies, accrediting bodies, and risk management—to avoid lawsuits • Patient confusion regarding paperwork • Patient time devoted to managing paperwork		X	X
5. Parking	• Unavailable or not within easy access • Limited handicapped parking. • Facilities charge for parking	X	X	

6. Geographical inconvenience	• Long distance travel required, especially for patients in rural areas • Medical facilities often not in proximity to laboratories and other diagnostic services	X		
7. Service hours inconvenience (i.e., limited service availability at night and on weekends)	When physician offices are closed • Patients may end up in the emergency room • Patients may forgo necessary medical care • Patients may self-diagnose and self-treat if they cannot see their physician	X	X	X
8. Cost of care, especially the out-of-pocket costs	• Insurance premiums increase with consumer portion expanding • Deductibles increase • Costs continue to increase along with add-on's such as co-pays and co-insurance • Increased costs may deter patients from seeking necessary care	X		X
9. Communication breakdowns even within the same unit or office	Because most facilities and offices do not have electronic record systems • Redundant requests for information • Patient records are incomplete or do not have up-to-date information relative to prescriptions • Inconsistent care instructions between providers and patients • Inaccurate communication of billing information among providers, insurers, and patients	X	X	X

10. No one-stop shopping—so it is time consuming as patients must visit various offices and businesses during the care process (pharmacy, physician's office, separate lab, etc.)	• Fragmentation of care • Lack of integration among providers and facilities • Patients must spend extra travel and waiting time with visits to a variety of facilities • Patients feel as if no one considers the value of their time spent in obtaining care at multiple locations	X	X	X

- Insured as well as uninsured adults perceived a need for major change. Only 16 percent of the respondents say the health care system works relatively well with only minor changes needed.
- Thirty percent reported that it is difficult or very difficult to get an appointment with a doctor the same or next day when sick.
- Sixty percent reported that it is difficult or very difficult to get care on nights, weekends, or holidays.
- Fifty-six percent reported that there were problems of coordination among providers if multiple doctors are involved in the care process.
- Seventy-three percent reported difficulty getting timely access to their doctor.
- Twenty-eight percent reported administrative hassles related to medical bills and insurance.
- Overwhelming proportions of the respondents (88–96 percent) support more accessible, coordinated, and well-informed care.
  - One doctor responsible for coordinating care
  - Place to go besides ER on nights and weekends
  - Easy access to your own medical records
  - All doctors have easy access to your medical records
  - You have quality information for different providers
  - You have cost information for different providers
- According to 86–89 percent of respondents, it is very important for doctors to use electronic medical records, access your test results, and share information electronically with other doctors.

PROBLEMS IN GETTING APPOINTMENTS

John and Mary are a married couple who have just moved to a Midwestern state. They did a scientific search to identify a primary care physician by consulting Best Doctors in America. *After identifying the best doctors in internal medicine and family practice in the metropolitan area, they began to search to find the perfect primary care physician. There were seven doctors listed in those specialties in the reference. After calling each one, they found that two had retired or were no longer in practice, others were not taking new patients, and the remainder did not accept their insurance. They have not yet found a primary care physician.*

A major reason most Americans have difficulty in getting appointments is that there is a shortage of primary care physicians, which is well-known and increasing. Most new physicians enter one of the specialties since they finish medical school with significant debt that they need to repay as soon as possible and specialists earn higher income than primary care physicians. In addition, many primary care physicians are aging and retiring from the profession.

The result is that most Americans do not have a primary care physician and have difficulty getting appointments for primary care services. Those lacking insurance often use the hospital emergency room, and insured patients often have to wait months for the next available appointment. The result is that most Americans receive most of their health care services on an episodic basis.

Primary care physicians usually avoid Medicaid patients and some also avoid Medicare patients, putting an increased burden on overwhelmed hospital emergency rooms. Many patients avoid contact with the health care system as long as possible and allow problems to become cumulative so that multiple interventions are needed by the time the patient is seen and assessed. The impact of all of the above on access is self-evident. Patients have difficulty getting appointments, postpone necessary care, and tend to experience multiple complications by the time care is received.

LONG WAITS FOR SERVICES

Charles is a professor at a major Southeastern university and academic medical center. Recently, a mole he had always had on his chest became enlarged and annoying. At the urging of his wife, he made an appointment at the dermatology clinic of the medical school. The dermatologist examined the mole, indicated it was probably benign (later confirmed), and removed it during the initial visit. Since some sutures were used, she scheduled a follow-up visit for Charles to have his sutures removed.

When Charles arrived for his follow-up appointment two weeks later, the outside temperature was 95 degrees. After arriving and signing in

10 minutes early for his 1 PM appointment, he waited 30 minutes and was then called in to an examining room. A medical student intern then asked him to remove his shirt and told him the dermatologist would be in shortly. The temperature in the examining room was 65 degrees, which was quite a change from the outdoor temperature. Charles began shivering and looking at his watch. At 2:15 he put his shirt back on, but the dermatologist had still not arrived. No one provided any information or explanation concerning the delay as he shivered in the cold examining room alone. Finally, at 3 PM he left the examining room and reemerged into the hot, humid outdoors with his sutures still intact and no evaluation of the healing process.

The current health care system and its providers do not value the consumers' time. If the health care insurers had to reimburse their enrollees for the time value of their time spent waiting for health services, costs would be much higher in the short run, but waiting times would be significantly lower in the long run. From the provider and insurer perspective, consumer time has no value since it is not reimbursable. Money drives the system and consumer time is not valued or reimbursed. The result is economizing on provider time (which is reimbursed) and ignoring the time value of patient time.

Patient waiting time could be reduced if there were a large number of primary care clinics located in proximity to where people live staffed by nurses, nurse practitioners, and physician assistants. Employer health clinics and retail health clinics offer models for how patient waiting times might be reduced in the future.

PATIENTS SPEND LITTLE TIME WITH PHYSICIANS

Emily visited her physician because she periodically has a pain in her lower left side that is often accompanied by some nausea and vomiting as well. Her appointment was scheduled for 10:00 AM, with instructions to arrive 15 minutes ahead of time to complete paperwork. Emily arrived at 9:45. At 10:00, she was given some forms to complete for insurance purposes and to comply with regulations for privacy. She was also given a patient history form to update her medical record. At 10:30, Emily was weighed and vital signs were taken. At 10:45, Emily was shown to the exam room and asked to put on a gown. At 11:15, fully 90 minutes after arriving at the office, Emily met with her physician. The physician apologized profusely for the delay and proceeded to ask Emily to describe her problem. At 11:21, the physician was finished with Emily. The physician suspects possible diverticulitis and wrote Emily a referral to a *gastroenterologist. At 11:30 AM, Emily entered a line of patients who were waiting to pay their bills, make future appointments, and pick up prescriptions and referrals. At 11:45, Emily paid her share of the bill, a co-pay of $20, and departed the physician's office. Of the two hours Emily spent in the physician's office, only 6 minutes were spent with the physician. Emily still does not feel well and now must wait to see a gastroenterologist.*

Patients are stressed when visiting their physicians because they perceive time pressures. The physician always seems to be in a hurry, having just left one patient and preparing to move on to the next. The physician enters the room and greets the patient while reading a paper or computer file of notes that document the patient's history. Then the physician might flip to results of laboratory or other clinical work and diagnostic tests while simultaneously asking questions of the patient or nodding silently in response to what is being heard or read.

The physician may not even look at the patient or lay hands on the patient during the visit. As the physician departs, the hand is extended, sometimes with a prescription, sheet of billing information for the front desk, and perhaps a sheet of information about the patient's disease. Just outside the examining room door, the physician is heard rapidly dictating physician notes for that visit or keying them into a computer program. Often when patients get to the billing area, they learn more details of what occurred during the visit, especially if there is a need to schedule a referral visit to a specialist or order a diagnostic test.

Why do physicians spend so little time with patients? The answer is the physician's time has a cash value and that cash value is critical to the facility's financial survival. Physicians are the most expensive health care professional. They represent the most highly trained and educated occupation in health care and, as such, their time is billed at a much higher rate than that of nurses and other health professionals. Subsequently, patients might wait an hour to see a physician, but end up with only an actual five minute visit because of the cost of a physician's time. Because specialty physicians bill at a higher rate than primary care doctors, their time spent with a patient is that much more expensive.

In the 1990s, managed care focused attention on the physician's contribution to overall productivity. Because physician time is the most expensive input, a patient visit was stratified to correlate with reimbursement levels that reflected acuity of care and resource usage, from routine to expanded care. For example, a routine patient visit might range from level one to level five, with level one representing the basic care and level five more complex care. Therefore, a level one visit for a new patient might involve a healthy 20-year-old with few complaints. A level five visit might involve a patient with more complex problems such as multiple chronic illnesses, including arthritis, diabetes, and heart disease.

A patient visit of 10 to 12 minutes consists of 5 to 7 minutes for meeting with the patient and the remaining time dedicated to physician notes for the medical record, writing prescriptions and referrals, and any other paperwork to document the visit. Despite recommendations by media and experts, which suggest patients bring "lists" of questions for the physician, there is little time available to explore much during a 5 to 7 minute visit. Today, it is not uncommon to find that physician offices post notices limiting patients to a specified number of questions or complaints. For example, a dermatologist's office might post a notice in the waiting area informing patients that they may only ask the doctor three dermatology questions during the visit. Additional questions would require scheduling an extra visit.

In addition, suggestions for patients to bring a friend or relative along to take notes and ensure that the patient's questions are answered might work better in theory than in practice. First, patient exam rooms have gotten smaller over the years and usually seat two people: the patient and the doctor. There is little room for additional guests. Second, the doctor is on a schedule that dictates seeing a certain number of patients during the workday. The patient's visit cannot be expanded for additional questions because there is no room in the schedule to accommodate such changes. In fact, there is usually little if any room on the schedule for walk-ins or patients with urgent care needs. Gone are the days when physician offices promised to "work" a sick patient into the schedule. Nowadays, if patients are sick and do not have a scheduled appointment, they are advised to go the emergency department.

Many physicians no longer accept Medicaid or Medicare patients because of their low reimbursement rates. And physicians who continue to accept Medicare patients frequently limit the visit to a single chronic disease, thereby requiring the patient to schedule multiple visits to address new or further problems. One elderly patient complained to her physician that it was difficult to schedule additional visits. She lived by herself and had to ask her granddaughter to take off work to drive her to the physician's office. The physician's office staff explained that scheduling additional visits was the only way the physician could continue to see Medicare patients. The patient was advised to find another doctor if this arrangement was unsuitable.

The physician's time is predetermined by payers such as insurers and the government through its public programs, Medicare or Medicaid. In order to maximize productivity, physician practices may hire an advanced practice nurse such as a nurse practitioner or a physician assistant to "work up" the patient prior to being seen by the physician. Both of these occupations are billed at a lower rate than the physician and consequently they can spend more time with the patient. This advance work reduces the time that the physician must spend with the patient.

In some cases, the nurse practitioner or physician assistant may conduct the entire patient visit so that the patient is never seen by the physician. For example, a physician assistant may perform routine skin cancer screenings or a nurse practitioner may conduct a gynecological exam, including a pap smear. In both cases, these health professionals are technically under physician supervision, but the physician is not physically present for the visit.

Why do physicians spend so little time with patients? It does not seem to be the patient's preference, and it is doubtful that physicians enjoy rushing from patient to patient. In the 1960s and 1970s, physicians had offices within their practices. Patients sat in an office with the physician's diplomas on the wall and medical books on shelves. Physicians spent time with patients in these offices if only to give them comfort and encouragement with a challenging diagnosis such as diabetes or heart disease. During the actual office visit, physicians laid hands on the patient and created a connection between the two.

The physician-patient relationship has been the cornerstone of American medicine, but over the years cost containment efforts have contributed to an erosion of that relationship. Physicians who have experienced the intimacy of the physician-patient relationship are retiring or retired. Physicians who have just entered the workforce after the advent of managed care or who are in training to do so are unaware of how physicians previously related with patients and the time spent with them during a visit. So when patients complain about limited time spent with the physician, some physicians are confounded by the complaint, especially those who are new to the practice of medicine. Older patients, however, are dissatisfied because their past experience with the health care system was more personal. Sick patients visit a physician to get better. They want their disease diagnosed, and they want recommendations for treatment. If that cannot be accomplished in five to seven minutes, patients feel shortchanged and justified with their complaints.

ADMINISTRATIVE PAPERWORK

Carol discovers a lump on one breast during a self-examination. She had already had breast cancer 20 years earlier and immediately became concerned. After identifying oncologists in her local area and talking to a number of other women, she selected an oncologist and made an appointment for an examination. The oncologist recommended surgical removal of the tumor followed by a biopsy and further treatment if the biopsy indicated malignancy. The biopsy came back positive and the oncologist recommended chemotherapy since radiation had previously been used on that breast 20 years earlier.

Carol followed the oncologist's advice: a surgeon removed the tumor, and she followed that up with chemotherapy visits each week for two months. Her mailbox substantively became full of statements from the hospital, the surgeon, and the oncologist. Also, separate statements were submitted by the insurance company. It was never clear what bills had or had not been paid by the insurer, what bills would be paid in the future, and what bills would not be reimbursable at all.

Managing of the paperwork became a full-time job since it typically required follow-up phone calls to the offices of the hospital, the surgeon, the oncologist, and the health insurer. No one was coordinating the paperwork, and so Carol had the job of identifying what had been paid, what might be paid, and what would not be paid. The phone calls involved being kept on hold for long periods of time, explaining and re-explaining the situations and specifics to multiple individuals, responding to denials, appealing decisions, paying bills, and investing enormous amounts of personal time in the process.

The administrative burden of our nonsystem of health services burdens all stakeholders including patients. Documentation is required for reimbursement purposes rather than to ensure quality care. Multiple paperwork systems exist, and they are not integrated with one another. The patient is asked to provide the same information over and over again for different providers and insurers. Statements are sent to patients by insurers and providers that are unclear in terms of whether the patient is being asked to pay the whole bill, part of the bill (a co-payment), or wait to see if the insurer pays the bill. Widely different payment rates apply to different patients.

The goal of all insurers (for-profit and nonprofit) is to generate a surplus of revenue over costs (i.e., reimbursements) on a consistent basis. Toward that end, insurers constantly change their panels and networks of providers, and contract out some services with a constantly changing panel of contractors, some of whom are in-network and some of whom are not. A consumer with a major or chronic health problem is forced into managing the whole process since there is no integration among providers or between insurers and providers. Reimbursement is routinely denied if any errors are detected and/or if the coverage is questionable. Even if the reimbursement is eventually approved, the time and effort required by the patient (and sometimes the provider) to achieve eventual approval makes the process costly and frustrating.

PARKING

John has been having some prostate problems, and his physician wants him to have an MRI to assist in confirming the diagnosis. The MRI will be performed at a facility that is adjacent to the hospital. John's appointment for the MRI is 10:00 AM. John arrives to find the hospital lots full as well as the parking garages. At 10:00, John is still driving around looking for parking. He uses his cellular phone to call the facility, and they suggest that he try looking for parking on the side streets. John does this and succeeds in finding a metered parking spot. It takes John a good 15 minutes to walk from his car to the facility. By this time it is 10:45, and his time slot has been given to someone else. The staff manages to work John into the schedule for 11:45. He returns to his car at 1:30 PM only to find that the meter has expired and his car has been ticketed.

As cities and suburbs grow more populated, parking is problematic. However, one expects parking to be less challenging at a health care facility, which deals with many patients who are ill, injured, or handicapped. Yet those who visit hospitals and other health facilities find crowded lots and few handicapped parking spots. In addition, often there are parking fees levied on patients and their visitors. This is especially true if the facilities are in urban areas or highly trafficked suburbs where parking is at a premium. In the past, hospitals and physician practices may have offered to validate patient parking. However, with cost controls and declining reimbursements, validated parking is less common these days. Some hospitals offer seniors a discount on the parking fees, but seniors either must apply for or in some cases purchase a reduced fee pass in advance.

Some of the larger hospitals offer remote lot parking, similar to airports. In these cases, shuttle vans and minibuses pick up the patients or visitors and deposit them at the hospital's entrance. However, there are waits for the shuttle buses and inclement weather to contend with, much like the airport parking. In some cases, there is a charge for the shuttle service. Some hospitals also offer "valet" parking to minimize the inconvenience, but valet service is not without its drawbacks, including waiting times, fees, and service limitations. Valet service in many cases is restricted to weekdays and working hours. Usually the number of valet parking slots is limited. If the valet slots are full, the patient must either wait in a queue for one to open or look to park elsewhere.

Because many outpatient facilities and physician offices are in proximity to hospitals, patients who visit these facilities can find parking there is limited as well. When the lots fill up, these patients compete for metered or on-street parking that is restricted by time limits. If a patient's visit runs long, which often happens, the patient likely will find a parking ticket. Some facilities might offer patients access to parking in the hospital parking garage across the street. There may or may not be a cost involved, but either way it requires the patient to walk some distance just to have access to parking.

Why is parking a problem? Most health care facilities are not designed with customer parking or convenient access to the facility in mind. Outpatient surgery clinics should have more than 10 percent of their parking spots dedicated to handicapped parking along with areas for dropping off and picking up patients. Few clinics or hospitals think in terms of true parking amenities for their patients. They might believe so, but patients arriving and departing in wheelchairs or on crutches or in their last trimester of pregnancy can be physically challenged to gain entrance to the facility from the parking lot. And charging for parking that is not convenient only adds to patient dissatisfaction.

Patients with emergencies may encounter problems with parking. Signs and directions to the emergency department are often not in plain view from the parking lots. Furthermore, there usually are no designated parking spots for patients seeking emergency care. When someone is traveling to the hospital for an emergency, the last thing they need to think about should be finding a parking spot. Drivers who abandon their cars in restricted areas in front of the emergency room return to find that their vehicle has been towed.

Why inconvenience patients and their families with parking? If women are seeking treatment at a facility for breast cancers, why confront them with parking problems? Shouldn't the parking needs of patients come first? Apparently not, because a drive through most lots and garages shows that the good spots, those nearest the facility and/or elevators, are reserved for top administrators, including physician administrators. Some facilities also reserve the close-in spaces for their employees. Even suppliers have dedicated parking spaces at some facilities. When patient satisfaction surveys report problems with parking, does anyone read them? When CEOs and other top health care executives are surveyed, their top concerns are always financial, especially reimbursement. Patient parking problems just do not make it to the top of the list.

GEOGRAPHICAL INCONVENIENCE

The Redding Family lives in a suburb outside of a major metropolitan city in the Midwest. The Reddings have access to primary care medicine in their suburban town, but for specialty care, including diagnostic testing, they are required to drive two hours to a nearby city. One of their children, eight-year-old Ralph, has a rare lung condition that requires the care of a pulmonologist. Ralph has monthly scheduled appointments and frequently undergoes respiratory testing prior to the appointment. Ralph's mother and father take turns driving him to his appointments so they will not use up all of their annual leave.

Health care facilities are not located for the geographical convenience of the consumer. Hospitals are usually built where land is less expensive. Sometimes, hospitals are built adjacent to a university and its medical college so that medical students and faculty have quick access to hospital facilities. Physician offices are often situated near hospitals, especially when physicians are specialists. Having an office nearby is particularly convenient for specialty physicians who have hospitalized patients. These doctors can conduct their patient reviews during rounds and quickly return to their offices for their regular patient visits. Physician offices also tend to be located where the rents or land are affordable. Few physicians select office space based on access to public transportation.

Patients seem to drive everywhere for their care, especially those who live in small towns and rural areas. Patients with chronic conditions often have to schedule multiple visits with a variety of providers. This means driving across town to see some doctors and going downtown to see others. If specialty care is required, patients may end up near the hospital or in another city altogether. When a physician leaves town, his patients may be transferred to another provider who is in a location that is much less convenient to the patient. The patient must then decide whether to attempt to find another doctor who is nearby or drive a considerable distance to the new physician's office.

And physicians change hospitals, too, often because of insurers. Insurers negotiate steep discounts with hospitals, and for the physicians to stay in network, they often are required to shift their patients to different hospitals. Furthermore, patients discover that their insurers can add or drop physicians and facilities with little notice and with little consideration of the convenience of the consumer.

One clinical laboratory was dropped by an insurer. This laboratory was located next to a group of university clinics and physician offices, which was convenient for patients who could have their lab work done and walk down the hall to see their physicians afterward. The new laboratory selected by the insurer was a 20 minute drive from the clinics and physician offices. In addition to the drive, the laboratory was located in an older building with limited handicapped access.

TIME INCONVENIENCE IN TERMS OF ACTUAL SERVICE HOURS

Seven-year-old Susan had a history of bad earaches. She woke up on Saturday morning with the worst earache ever. She went immediately to her parent's bedroom and told them about it. Her mother called the pediatrician's office and left a voice mail message. An hour later, the call was returned by an operator for the answering service. The operator informed Susan's mother that the voice mail had been relayed to the physician, and he felt that Susan should be taken to the emergency department. Susan and her mom went to the emergency department at noon on Saturday. The emergency department was already at full capacity. They waited seven hours to be seen by a physician who prescribed an antibiotic and instructions to follow-up with their own physician on Monday.

The health care delivery system is not equipped to handle those who become ill in the evenings, during holidays, and on weekends. Doctors' office and clinical facilities are usually closed evenings and weekends. And when people do not feel well, especially if the discomfort is a sudden occurrence, they become worried and want to be seen by their doctor.

Nowadays, if a patient phones a doctor's office after working hours, they will more than likely encounter a recording. The recording instructs the patient that the doctor's office is closed, repeats the hours when the office is open, and advises the patient that in the case of an emergency to please hang up and call 911. For the patient who is doubled over with stomach pain, this recording is less than helpful. The patient will be reluctant to call 911 for what might be an upset stomach. Instead, the patient will lie awake all night with the pain and worry.

In the 1960s and early 1970s, family physicians would make house calls to see patients who became ill after hours. If patients became ill at 8 PM, they could phone the physician for advice and possibly a face-to-face visit. The physician might recommend coming into the office first thing the next morning, but if the physician felt it was necessary, he would set out to see the patient later that evening. In the 1960s and 1970s, physicians "worked" sick patients into their schedules and often stayed late at their offices to accommodate them.

Patients were not automatically referred to 911 calls or emergency departments for their complaints. They were seen by their family physicians for their colds, earaches, and stomach upsets. Sometimes physicians might use an answering service to handle calls that came in after they departed the office. However, if the patient had an emergency, the physician would take her call. New mothers especially benefited from knowing that they could always depend on their doctors to be available for their questions and concerns.

When sick patients call a physician's office during working hours today, they are most likely informed that the schedule is full for the next several weeks or months. Patients do not speak with the physician or even a physician substitute such as a nurse practitioner. Instead, patients are told by the receptionist that the doctor is booked for the next three weeks and if the patient feels he cannot wait for the appointment, the patient should proceed to the emergency department.

Most patients are not comforted with the receptionist's advice. If the patient is feeling extremely ill, he might proceed to the emergency department of a local hospital and wait to be seen. If the patient is in extreme pain upon arrival at the emergency department, he likely will remain in pain until he can be seen. Because there is a triage system in emergency medicine that prescribes treating the sickest patients first, patients with earaches and stomach pains will be among the last to be seen.

To attempt to manage the problem of patients getting sick after hours and on weekends, some insurers now offer a telephone evaluation service that is staffed by nurse practitioners. Patients may call a special 800 telephone number to get a telephonic assessment of their condition. For example, a patient may call on a Friday evening about a stomach pain. The nurse doing the assessment may decide that the pain is probably just an upset stomach and recommend some over-the-counter product. If the patient does not get better, however, he is advised to go to the emergency department and, of course, to follow up with his physician.

Physicians have been challenged by scheduling problems for some time now. Most physician scheduling is done for future appointments. For example, when a patient sees the physician for a routine physical exam, the patient simultaneously schedules the next visit for a future date. Eventually, the physician's calendar is full of future appointments for routine items such as immunizations and checkups.

There are alternative scheduling methods that would allow the physician to allocate time each day to accommodate sick patients. One method calls for the physician to "carve out" a specified number of hours each day for sick patients. However, physicians have been slow to adopt such methodologies, most likely because they fear patients will not show up to fill the slots, and they will lose revenue as a result. Therefore, physicians will likely continue to schedule "future" appointments at the expense of patients who are sick today. And patients will continue to self-diagnose and self-treat their health problems or seek care in emergency departments.

ESCALATING COSTS FOR THE SYSTEM AND THE CONSUMER

Helen's physician gave her the good news. She did not have ovarian cancer as originally suspected. She had some tumors, but they were not cancerous. Helen was very grateful to her physician and the hospital until she got her bill. Helen received a bill for anesthesia services that showed she had not used a network provider. Therefore, she was required to pay 60 percent of the bill instead of 20 percent. Helen called the hospital's billing office and argued that she had verified that the hospital was in the network. Unfortunately, no one had explained to Helen that some hospital services such as anesthesia were privately provided and not included in the network. Helen was responsible for paying the out-of-network charges for the anesthesia services.

Patients confront rising health care costs, including increases in the premium expense for health insurance and also escalating out-of-pocket costs. Patients complain about these increases, but who listens to them? Physicians and their office staff may empathize with patients, but they cannot alter the patient's insurance. Most physician offices and hospital billing departments do their best to advise patients, but these offices deal with too many different types of insurance to keep up-to-date on all changes. Consequently, patients are advised by posted and printed notices that it is the patient's responsibility to verify insurance matters.

Instead of advocating for patients and their concerns about cost escalations, physicians and hospitals often add to the problem by attempting to go after patients for additional monies. For example, some hospitals are charging facility fees when you visit your physician in a hospital setting such as a dermatology clinic instead of in his private office (Merrill, 2009). In addition, hospitals and physicians have attempted to obtain increased fees through something called balance billing. This occurs when patients are billed for the "balance" or difference between what the insurer determines is allowed for payment and the amount that was requested for payment by either the hospital or physician. Recently California enacted legislation to outlaw balance billing for emergency physicians. However, California hospitals and physicians protested that managed care organizations were engaging in underpayments of $1 billion to emergency departments for 2007 (Sorrel, 2009).

Patients can complain to their employers about rising out-of-pocket costs, especially concerns with premiums. In some cases employers can work with both employees and insurers to reduce premium costs, but usually such reductions involve eliminating some health benefits and increasing costs for others. For example, employers have eliminated healthy screening benefits such as cancer screenings to bring premium costs down. Or the insurer has increased the rates for additional family members. In some instances, insurers have reduced the prescription drug benefit or increased co-payment amounts.

Patients can complain directly to insurers, but insurers are hired by the employer. An employer will negotiate a contract with an insurer to provide employees with health care coverage. Just as employers focus on efficiency and keeping costs down, insurers look to satisfy employer demands by offering reduced health insurance costs. One way they attempt to do this is by increasing the out-of-pocket amount that patients must pay. Insurers increase this amount by using deductibles, co-payments (co-pays), co-insurance, and levying additional fees for service delivery outside of a prespecified network of providers, including physicians and facilities.

Patients have to meet the deductible amount before they are eligible for coverage. Deductibles can range from as low as $250 annually for an individual to $500 to $1,000 and beyond. There are family deductibles, too, so that expenses for a family can be aggregated and applied to a deductible. Much like automobile insurance, the amount of the deductible will correlate with the insurance premium. For example, higher deductibles usually correspond to lower premiums. But unlike automobile insurance, once the deductible is met for health care, there are additional limitations on what the health care insurer will pay. For example, if an individual has a $500 deductible and meets that amount, the health care insurer might thereafter pay only 80 percent of what they determine is an allowable amount for the service that is rendered. The patient will be responsible for the remaining 20 percent. This amount is referred to as co-pay.

Health insurers also now request payment of co-insurance, which is typically described as an additional amount that the insurer can add to the patient's bill. A decade earlier, the concept of co-insurance did not exist in health care; now it is fairly standard. There are no co-pays or co-insurance amounts used in conjunction with automobile or homeowner's insurance, making the health insurance industry unique in this respect.

Another factor that influences escalating costs is the insurer's use of the concept of networks to determine payments. Insurers have organized providers into networks. If the patient uses a network provider, either a physician or facility, the cost is less to the patient. If, however, the patient chooses to use a provider that is outside of the network, the cost to the patient increases, usually substantially. Health insurers have negotiated discounts with their provider networks, and they incentivize patients to use network providers to keep costs down. But patient choice in such matters is not always clear-cut.

For example, a patient can select a hospital and physician who are in the insurer's network only to discover that one of the hospital's services, such as pathology, which is required for a biopsy, is not. Many times, typical hospital-based services such as anesthesiology, pathology, and even emergency medicine are provided by private companies through contractual arrangements with the hospital. These private companies typically are not in the insurer's network because they are unwilling to discount their services. The patient who has need of these services has no choice but to pay the out-of-network rate, which is not discounted. Such matters have grown so complicated that even outpatient surgery centers advise patients to verify whether the facility charges, including the anesthesia service, are covered by their insurance.

If patients complain enough about an insurer, will the employer listen? It all depends. Employers need to save money on insurance costs in order to remain profitable and competitive. Many employers consider dropping health insurance altogether because of escalating costs. Even health care facilities are challenged by the cost of health insurance.

A sports medicine clinic had a meeting with employees and showed them the numbers. They would either have to lay off workers in order to continue to be able to offer health insurance or drop health insurance as a benefit. When confronted with these choices, the workers offered up a third alternative: increase employee out-of-pocket costs. In doing so, the employer's expense for coverage was reduced.

Because health care costs only increase, it is likely that many employers will find themselves in similar situations. It is also probable that employees will not voice complaints about increases in out-of-pocket expenses if it means their jobs or loss of coverage altogether. Whatever insurers do to reduce the employee's premium will be reflected in the health benefits that are offered. Because insurance companies are big business and their profits are widely reported, employees and their employers wonder why they must pay more.

COMMUNICATION BREAKDOWNS

Carleen is the wife of a faculty member in a small college town in the Southeast. She recently discovered a lump on her breast and went to see her local primary care physician. He referred her to a local surgeon who recommended removal of the tumor, a biopsy, and a radical mastectomy if it was malignant. She and her husband decided a second opinion was in order. She then called her primary care physician and requested a referral to an oncologist at the academic medical center 60 miles away. He said he did not know anyone there and assured her that the local surgeon was "the best."

She then researched oncologists nationally and found one of the best in the nation was at that medical center. She initiated a call to the medical center, found the number of the oncologist, called his office, and made an appointment without a referral. The oncologist was participating in a clinical trial which he suggested that Carleen join. This clinical trial involved the removal of the tumor followed by radiation treatment if the tumor was malignant. As it turned out, the tumor was malignant and Carleen followed a radiation regiment for six weeks. She did not suffer a recurrence of her breast cancer for many years. Communication between the oncologist and the primary care physician was nonexistent throughout this period.

One of the challenges the Obama administration would like to address is the lack of electronic medical records in health care. They believe that electronic medical records will enhance access and quality while reducing costs in the system. Whether or not these lofty goals are eventually achieved, there is no doubt that an integrated system of electronic medical records available to all stakeholders, including the patient, would be a tremendous improvement over what we have now.

The idea would be for each patient to have an electronic medical record that would be updated each time a service was received. In that way, all providers and insurers could access relevant information on the patient and paperwork would be significantly reduced for all. Obviously, we are nowhere near that situation at the time of this writing (2009). Among the most important impediments are the tremendous costs associated with this initiative as well as patient privacy concerns. Part of the stimulus money appropriated by Congress in 2009 was spent on enhanced electronic medical records.

Retailers such as Walmart have made some inroads. For example, Walmart announced plans to begin marketing an affordable digital health records system in 2009. This venture reflects a partnership of Walmart with high-tech companies, including Dell and eClinicalWorks (Lohr, 2009).

NO ONE-STOP SHOPPING

Robert has recently moved to a new area of the country and identified a potential primary care physician based on the recommendation of some close friends. Robert has recently visited his primary care physician, a doctor of osteopathic medicine, who has given him a rather superficial examination and asked him to gather additional information as a follow-up to this initial visit. The doctor indicated to Robert that no testing is done in his office or in the building in which his office is housed. He suggested that Robert needed a blood test to check for cholesterol and other health indicators. In addition, he suggested an EKG since Robert was more than 50 years of age and had never had an EKG.

Robert was told by the nurse that he needed to visit a testing lab 8 miles away for his blood test. Then he would need to schedule an appointment and go to another facility for his EKG. In both cases, he would have to retrieve the test results and bring them back to the primary care physician. Robert left with a fist full of paperwork and thought about the recommended follow-up visits he was asked to schedule. He then decided to not do those follow-up visits and continue looking for another primary care physician.

Just as consumers are asked to manage the avalanche of paperwork associated with their care, they are also asked to manage and coordinate a wide-range of providers. In most cases, as noted previously, these providers do not communicate accurately and comprehensively with one another. They only know what their patients tell them, and their information systems are not necessarily compatible with one another. All of this reflects the fact that patient time is not reimbursable and is considered "free."

In theory, primary care physicians coordinate care provided by all providers; however, as noted previously, most Americans do not have a primary care physician and even those who do, do not spend a lot of time with them or have all of their care coordinated. There may be a few academic medical centers where care is provided in one geographic location and coordinated among all of the providers in that system. However, this is the exception and not the rule.

CONCLUSION

Most Americans experience significant challenges and hassles in their attempts to receive necessary health services for themselves and their families. The system is unintegrated and uncoordinated. The burden of trying to put the pieces together falls on the patients themselves rather than the providers or insurers. For most Americans health services are episodic in nature and preventive care is practically nonexistent. The focus is on curative care, which is more expensive, and the result is mortality and morbidity in the United States that is no better than average relative to other developed countries. The question is whether retail medicine offers potential for alleviating these hassles, and if so, how this potential might be realized in the future.

REFERENCES

How, S. K. H., Shih, A., Lau, J., & Schoen, C. (2008). "Public views on U.S. health system organization: A call for new directions." The Commonwealth Fund. http://www.commonwealthfund.org/Content/Surveys/2008/The-Commonwealth-Fund-Survey-of-Public-Views-of-the-U-S–Health-Care-System–2008.aspx (accessed April 8, 2009).

Lohr, S. (March 11, 2009). "Wal-Mart Plans to market digital health records system." *The New York Times.* Retrieved March 12, 2009, from http://www.nytimes.com/2009/03/11/business/11record.html.

Merrill, K. (March 10, 2009). "Some hospitals charging facility fees for care." Retrieved March 31, 2009, from wbztv.com/local/hospital.facility.fee.2.955941.html.

Sorrel, A. L. (January 26, 2009). "California's high court bans balance billing." amednews.com. Retrieved on April 12, 2009, from http://www.ama-assn.org/amednews/2009/0126.htm.

Chapter 4

Retail-Based Health Care Clinics: A "Disruptive Innovation"

Retail-based health care clinics (sometimes called convenient care clinics) offer a limited number of primary care diagnostic and treatment services for common medical conditions as well as preventive and wellness health services (Lin, 2008). These retail clinics are located in convenient locations where consumers shop, such as general merchandise retailers, drugstores, and grocery stores. They are usually staffed by family nurse practitioners and/or physician assistants. These medical professions can and do write prescriptions where appropriate. Most in-store retail clinics provide a prominent list of prices for all services to address issues of price transparency.

The first retail clinic opened in 2000, and today there are more than 1,100 clinics operated by more than 25 companies and health systems nationally (Convenient Care Association, 2008). Such clinics constitute a small but rapidly growing segment of the health care marketplace. However, retail clinics should grow rapidly as a result of consumer preferences for accessibility, convenient locations, reliability, and lower prices.

Innovations such as retail clinics are driven by necessity. They emerged and proliferated in response to the growth of obstacles that have hindered or prevented the delivery of primary health care services to Americans. Among these obstacles have been the convergence of overcrowded emergency departments, the growing shortage of primary care physicians, escalating insurance costs, and less insurance coverage for many Americans.

In response to these obstacles, large American retailers, such as Walmart, have identified an opportunity and engaged in what has been termed "strategic entrepreneurship." Strategic entrepreneurship typically involves a large corporation that devotes part of its resources to exploiting new market opportunities not addressed by current participants in the market (Fottler & Malvey, 2007).

These "strategic entrepreneurs" then develop what has been termed a "disruptive innovation" to address the unmet need and enhance their own financial returns. The term "disruptive innovation" was originated by Clayton Christensen and his colleagues in a 2000 *Harvard Business Review* article (Christensen et al., 2000). He and his colleagues noted that such innovations may disrupt whole industries because they enable less skilled employees to perform functions previously performed by more skilled and more expensive specialist employees. The newer disruptive innovations are also performed in settings that are more convenient and less costly.

In-store retail clinics may be more than a disruptive innovation to the health care delivery system. They have the potential to be a catalyst for improving health care access and affordability for primary care services in this country. As such, they should be viewed as a step in the maturation process for health systems that are focused on creating more consumer-friendly health care options (PricewaterhouseCoopers, 2005). They are not the singular solution to all of the nation's health care challenges, but rather, one step in the incremental improvement of our health care delivery system.

CONCEPTUAL FRAMEWORK

Strategic Entrepreneurship

Corporations currently entering or already in the retail health clinic market have exhibited behavior that has been characterized as strategic entrepreneurship, which combines the concepts of strategic management and entrepreneurship. Entrepreneurship is "the identification and exploitation of previously unexploited opportunities" (Hitt, Ireland, Camp, & Sexton, 2001), which often "involves bundling resources and deploying them to create new organizational and industry configurations" (Schoonhoven & Romanelli, 2001). The opportunity to exploit entrepreneurial opportunities to form sustainable competitive advantage is available to all organizations, large and small. However, many fail to motivate their managers to pursue entrepreneurial opportunities (Day & Wendler, 1998).

Both the seeking of new opportunities (i.e., entrepreneurship) and the seeking of competitive advantage within existing markets (i.e., strategic management) are required to create wealth (Ireland, Hitt, & Sirmon, 2003). One without the other is insufficient (Amit & Zott, 2001; Hitt & Ireland, 2000). Consequently, some combination of both is important in predicting the potential success of new ventures.

Historically, new companies have focused on identifying potential new markets but have been less focused and less successful in developing and sustaining their initial competitive advantages over time. Alternatively, more mature companies are better at strategic management but less successful in identifying and taking advantage of new market opportunities (Ireland, Hitt, & Sirmon, 2003). Organizations integrating entrepreneurship and strategy (i.e., strategic entrepreneurs) seek new opportunities to disrupt an industry's competitive environment to create new markets.

Disruptive Innovations

The organization must apply creativity and develop innovation to implement the process of strategic entrepreneurship. Schumpeter (1934) noted that innovation involves creating new combinations of labor and capital. The result may be the production of new goods and services, new processes for creating or using a service, new channels of distribution, or the development of new organizational structures. Innovation is linked to successful performance because innovations create new value for customers (Kluge, Meffert, & Stein, 2000). Disruptive innovation produces revolutionary change such as new services. Sustaining innovation creates incremental change and results from learning how to exploit the organization's existing capabilities and resources. It is often focused on development of new processes rather than development of new goods and services (Tushman & O'Reilly, 1996).

By contrast, disruptive innovation is the result of learning how to identify and exploit market opportunities by combining resources in new ways. These combinations may create new capabilities that, in turn, may create competitive advantage through new market development and new service delivery models. (Christensen,

Johnson, & Dann, 2002). These new models typically conflict with existing models and offer consumers new services or new methods of accessing existing services. Examples of disruptive innovations include Internet banking, low-fare airlines, online stock trading, and supply-chain innovations at Walmart (Charitou & Markides, 2003).

However, simpler alternatives to costly health services are resisted by the beneficiaries of the more costly service delivery model (Christensen et al., 2000; 2004). Such resistance to less expensive options by established organizations is common and understandable. This is not in the interest of either patients or the industry itself. If the industry is open to market forces and disruptive innovations that threaten existing ways of providing services, the result will be a higher quality of care together with lower costs for these services over time.

There are two types of disruptive innovations: "low-end" and "new-market" (Christensen et al., 2004). Low-end disruptive innovations deliver low-price alternatives to customers who are overshot by existing offerings. New-market disruptive innovations create new growth by making it easier for people to do something that previously required deep-end, expensive expertise. Retail clinics are *both* low-end and new-market disruptive innovations.

Since they are less expensive, easier to understand, and more user friendly than existing products or services, they typically begin now by addressing the service requirements of less demanding customers. Such disruptive innovations have caused many of history's best companies to plunge into crisis and ultimately to fail. This phenomenon of overshooting the needs of average customers and creating the potential for disruption quite accurately describes the health care industry today (Christensen et al., 2000).

Our major health care institutions have generally provided higher levels of care than is required by most patients. Most health care issues are relatively straightforward problems. However, our medical schools have prepared doctors to do much more than what is required for the diagnosis and treatment of most of these problems. Very little of our medical research funding is spent on training primary care doctors to provide basic services in ways that are simpler, more convenient, and less costly (Christensen et al., 2000).

Retail clinics are a disruptive innovation in the health care industry because they address routine health needs, are located in convenient locations, provide quick access, do not require appointments, are relatively low priced, and provide services during evening and weekend hours. These clinics fundamentally change how service is delivered because the point of care is more accessible and the provider is typically not a physician (Tu & Cohen, 2008).

Disruptive innovation has created major improvements in clinical outcomes and quality of life for most Americans. There are two options for addressing this dilemma. First, we might ask complex, high-cost institutions and their costly specialized physicians to move down-market and provide more basic care. This would obviously be an expensive option. A second option is to allow less costly professionals such as nurse practitioners and physician assistants to incrementally add more sophisticated services over time and provide them in less costly settings.

Non-physician practitioners are able to provide more complex services than they currently do in most settings. Nurse practitioners, for example, can be utilized in providing services that previously were done only by physicians. These clinicians are now able to provide diagnosis and treatment for simple conditions that previously would have required the training and judgment of a physician. However, many states impose constraints on these services by state law.

The regulations of many states to prohibit nurses from making diagnoses or prescribing medications they are trained to provide leads to inefficiency and higher costs than would otherwise be the case. The result is that primary care physicians often provide services that could be supplied by others at a lower cost. Such encounters adversely affect convenience, clinical quality, and the satisfaction levels of both patients and the physicians themselves.

Health care reform proposals today fall into three types of solutions: ask patients to consume fewer health care services and/or providers to become more efficient in order to contain costs; impose reimbursement controls that force expensive providers to become more efficient; and provide subsidies for the health care services of targeted subgroups. These proposals do not address the fundamental challenges that the health care system faces today because they are not consumer-driven.

Health care reform will require the creation of new institutions, such as retail clinics, that are able to deliver primary care services to most patients in a high-quality, but less costly, manner. These clinics are evolving and restructuring over time to better meet the needs of patient populations. Encouraging, supporting, and removing impediments to their development makes more sense than attempting to modify existing health care organizations that were designed to respond to the environmental requirements of the past.

DESCRIPTION OF RETAIL-BASED HEALTH CARE CLINICS

This section will provide a description of retail-based health care clinics, including consumer perceptions, the types of services they provide, providers of these services, contractors, and targeted populations.

Retail health clinics are located in a wide variety of retail settings including supermarkets, drugstores, and large retailers such as Walmart, Walgreens, Publix Supermarket, and CVS. They offer basic primary care services such as preventive services (i.e., physical exams) and treatment for simple health problems such as the common cold, lacerations, broken or sprained bones, and mild infections. They typically are open weekend and evening hours and employ either nurse practitioners or physician assistants. Their prices are typically lower than those in alternative settings and are prominently displayed (Scott, 2006). They have grown rapidly in recent years from 60 in 2006 to 1,100 in mid-2008 (Scott, 2008).

Insured patients and those with a regular physician may use retail clinics due to their convenient locations and the availability of walk-in visits. This is particularly likely when their service needs revolve around basic primary care services (curative or preventative). Patient co-payments are the same for a physician's office visit as for a retail clinic visit.

For the uninsured, however, clinics could provide a less expensive and more accessible option than other alternatives such as physician office visits or hospital emergency departments. Most lower-income people have less flexible work schedules with little or no time off. For them, the availability of extended hours may be crucial for their accessing the health care system at all. One recent study found that retail clinics serve a clientele that is underserved by primary care physicians (Mehrotra et al., 2008).

Consumer Perceptions of Retail Health Clinics

Between April 2007 and January 2008 a national survey was conducted using a national telephone sample of 9,400 families with approximately 18,000 people (Center for Studying Health System Change, 2007).

First, this survey indicated that consumers have had relatively little direct experience with retail clinics. Only 2.3 percent of consumers polled had actually used a retail health clinic at all, of which 73 percent had health insurance and 27 percent did not. Sixty-eight percent had insurance pay part or all of the cost, whereas 33 percent did not have insurance or had insurance that did not pay any of the costs.

Second, the most common services received at retail clinics included:

- New illness or symptoms—48 percent
- Prescription renewal—47 percent
- Vaccination—23 percent
- Care of ongoing chronic condition—18 percent
- Physical exam—14 percent
- Other—5 percent

Third, reasons for respondents' preferences for retail clinics over other alternatives were as follows:

- Convenient clinic hours—64 percent
- Convenient location—62 percent
- No appointment required—53 percent
- Lower cost—48 percent
- No usual source of care—34 percent

However, a Harris Interactive online survey among a national sample of 2,245 adults in 2007 indicated that only 5 percent of U.S. households had received services at a retail health clinic (Harris Interactive, 2007). Most of the surveyed adults had never experienced a retail clinic, and consequently were responding to their *perceptions* of such clinics.

Results were as follows:

- Seventy-eight percent agreed that retail clinics provide busy people with a fast and easy way to access basic medical services.
- Seventy-five percent agree that clinics can provide low-cost basic services to people who otherwise might not be able to afford care.

- Eighty-three percent agree that clinics can provide medical services to people when doctors' offices are closed.

However, 75 percent agree they would be worried serious medical problems might not be diagnosed and 71 percent worry about staff qualifications in clinics not run by physicians.

Retail Clinic Providers and Contractors

Table 4.1 provides a summary listing of existing retail health care clinics, where they can be found, and common as well as distinguishing attributes. It is evident from this summary that retailers are essentially testing a variety of clinic models. As such, they are carefully evaluating the potential of these clinics to increase the foot traffic in their stores and ultimately their revenues. This is also an example of implementing a low cost, albeit disruptive innovation. None of these retailers have invested so much in retail clinics that they do not have the flexibility to exit the health care business if it does not enhance their store revenues.

The clinics are not owned, staffed, or managed by retailers. Rather, retailers are outsourcing and leasing space to subcontractors who function as the clinic proprietors. These subcontractors typically are entirely responsible for clinic operations, including liability insurance. Walmart, for example, has partnered with Inter-Fit Health and other clinic providers (Spencer, 2005). They need to partner with outside clinic providers as a result of federal legislation that bans "self-referrals." This means that retailers that offer pharmacy services cannot run their own clinics. Walmart hopes that these new services will boost pharmacy business as customers fill prescriptions, as well as purchase other goods and services, while they are in the store.

Ownership of the in-store clinics that are found in retail establishments varies widely. Physician entrepreneurs have developed some clinics. Other clinics are owned or capitalized by equity investment firms. For example, Revolution Health Group (RHG) has capitalized RediClinics. These are retail-based health clinics that are located inside popular retail outlets such as Walmart stores (PRN Newswire, 2005). A few retail health care clinics are actually owned and managed by not-for-profit health care systems such as Aurora QuickCare, which is owned by Aurora Health Care, a Wisconsin health care system whose goals are aimed at increasing access to health care for its communities (Rice, 2005).

TABLE 4.1   Basic Medical Care Clinics Operating in "Retail" Establishments

Clinic Name	Current "Retail" Locations	Summary Information and Web Source Information
Solantic	23 clinics in Florida	• One of four clinic entrepreneurs selected to be used as a model by Walmart • A mixture of freestanding clinics and clinics inside Walmart Supercenters • Includes physicians on site • See http://www.solantic.com
RediClinics	75 locations in Arkansas, Indiana, Oklahoma, New York, and Texas	• One of four clinic entrepreneurs selected to be used as a model by Walmart • Currently "cash" business, but is considering third-party payments • Fixed price menu for all diagnostic tests ($45) • See http://www.rediclinic.com/
MinuteClinics	Selected Target stores, Cub supermarkets, and CVS pharmacy stores in Minnesota, Maryland, Florida, Georgia, Indiana, Kansas, North Carolina, Ohio, Tennessee, and Washington and in corporate settings and on University of Minnesota campus	• Has a strong national presence, operating more than 500 clinics mostly in CVS stores • Most of their business is third-party payment (90% of patients) • Commended by Clark Howard, national radio personality who promotes efforts to help consumers • Reported to compete with FastCare and MediMin • See http://www.minute clinic.com
Aurora QuickCare	10 clinics in Wisconsin Pharmacies and Piggly Wiggly supermarkets	• This is operated by a Non-Profit Health Care system, Aurora Health Care, which also includes traditional system components such as hospitals • See http://www.aurorahealth care.org

| Take Care Clinics | 300 Walgreens and Rite Aid stores in 32 cities | • Announced partnerships with the grocery store chain Albertsons Inc., Brooks Eckerd Pharmacy, and Rite Aid Corp.
• In "talks" with Walgreens
• See http://www.takecare health.com |
| The Little Clinic | 99 locations in 8 states | • Formerly known as FastCare, which was recently purchased by Solera Capital, a New York Equity Investment firm
• See http://www.thelittle clinic.com |

Note: Data for this table were developed from references used in this paper and the Web sources reported above.

Despite ownership differences, the retail health care clinics are very similar in nature. They offer fast access to common or basic health care services such as earaches, sore throat, immunizations, and preventive screenings. They are staffed by nurse practitioners, physician assistants, or advanced practice nurses who are authorized by law to see patients and prescribe medication in most states. Physician backup is available usually through telephone or email (Spencer, 2005).

Consequently, these clinics may serve as an entry point to the health care system because they provide referrals to those patients who do not have a primary care physician. All clinics offer extended hours, including evening hours and weekends. Typically no appointments are needed, and there is little waiting time. Clinic visits tend to be brief or about 15 minutes. Patients usually can use waiting time by shopping elsewhere in the store (Andrews, 2004; Rice, 2005; and Spencer, 2005).

Potential Impacts on Cost, Quality, and Access

Table 4.2 illustrates the potential impact on cost, quality, and access that retailers might have on delivery of basic health care services. Patients are expected to benefit because of convenience, cost, and enhanced access to basic medical services. In terms of costs, retailers represent reduced costs for third-party payers and patients alike. Most of the cost savings comes from efficiencies, such as using nurse practitioners instead of physicians.

TABLE 4.2   Potential Impact of Retail Clinics on Patients

Cost	Quality	Access
Positive		
Reduce cost by matching resources with patients' needs. Basic care for basic needs.	Assure quality through the use of standardized protocols (cookbook medicine) that are appropriate for basic care needs of patient.	Enhance access for all patients, especially the uninsured and underinsured because of affordability.
Reduce cost and boost productivity by using technology to enable less skilled workers to perform higher order functions.	Assure quality because if the patient's symptoms exceed diagnostic parameters, the patient is referred to a higher level of care—either an emergency department or family physician.	Enhance access because the number of locations for clinic visits is expanded. Also, most retail operations are located near public transportation.
Reduce cost by pressuring suppliers (i.e., subcontractors) to keep costs low.	Assure quality because continuity of care is established by trans-mitting (email or fax) patient's visit to the primary care physician.	Enhance access because the hours of operation are expanded and include late nights and weekends.
Reduce cost because of low fixed expenses such as office space, equipment, and furniture.	Assure quality because patients are seen by licensed and trained health professionals who are qualified to deliver basic health care services.	Enhance access because third-party payers increasingly are providing reim-bursement, including public programs such as Medicare.
Reduce cost because of ability to undercut competitors' prices.	Assure quality by making performance transparent.	Enhance access because the waiting time to be seen is minimal and appointments are not necessary.

Negative		
If patients abandon their primary care providers, they may end up with complications that require more expensive care.	Continuity of care may be affected if primary care providers are not integrated into the continuum of care.	If patients abandon their primary care providers, they may find that there is a waiting list to return, especially in areas where shortages already exist.
Patients may find themselves paying for care twice if they are referred to the emergency department.	Patients may self-diagnose an emergency condition as basic medical care.	Access to chronic care services may be jeopardized if patients mistakenly perceive that retail clinics are appropriate for chronic care needs.
Not all retail clinics accept insurance. Thus, patients may have to pay out of pocket for entire cost of visit.	Patient health and safety may be compromised if the in-store retail clinic does not have access to patient history.	Access to care may be compromised if the retail clinic changes subcontractors or consolidates clinics at all but a few locations.

The charges for services tend to be much lower than what would be expected in an emergency department or physician practice. A typical visit charge ranges between $25 and $60. This compares favorably with visits to other providers. For example, a primary care physician visit for basic services reportedly costs insurers $110 compared with the cost at a retail health care clinic, which is under $60. Consequently, insurers are supportive at this point (Spencer, 2005).

In addition, the clinic services are much less expensive compared with emergency room care. For example, a strep throat test costs $44 at MinuteClinics, which are found in Target, compared with $109 for a physician office visit, and $328 in the emergency department (Andrews, 2004). Some clinics operate as strictly "cash" businesses. Still others increasingly accept third-party payment.

Additionally, because of the low costs for most services, the uninsured and underinsured may also be able to access treatments for their health care needs. Enhanced access is also expected because the number of possible treatment locations will be expanded and hours of operations are extended to include nights and weekends. This will contribute to consumer convenience.

Quality of care has been the focal point of most concern and skepticism, especially by the physicians. However, consider that many people delay or postpone seeking care because it is not affordable or because they cannot get an appointment. Instead, they often self-diagnose and self-treat, using over-the-counter medications. Thus it would seem that a visit to a retail health care clinic would be preferable.

There are also complaints that these clinics are predominantly staffed by non-physician clinicians such as nurse practitioners, physician assistants, and advanced practice nurses. The rationale behind these complaints is that these providers are not as highly trained as physicians and as such are incapable of providing care of comparable quality. This is true in that physicians have more education and training than nurse practitioners, for example. But the reverse argument holds that physicians may be overeducated and overqualified to treat ear infections and other basic disorders. In this regard, their skill level does not correspond with the difficulty of the medical problem, and lower cost/lesser skilled providers such as physician assistants would have skills more aligned with the task requirements.

As a result of diagnostic and therapeutic technology improvements, both physician assistants and nurse practitioners are now able to proficiently diagnose and treat illnesses and oversee disease management. Additionally, because the cost of physician services is high relative to nurse practitioners, physicians are forced to see more patients over time. This is called *churning* and frequently means that because of the discrepancy in personnel costs, the physician can spend only a few minutes with a patient compared with a nurse practitioner (Christensen, Bohmer, & Kenagy, 2000).

Most of the retail health care clinics use standardized protocols and electronic medical records. In the case of MinuteClinics, which are located in Target stores, they reportedly invested $15 million in software that uses clinical protocols that have been established through medical research and endorsed by various physician associations. The clinics also offer physician backup through email or the telephone (Andrews, 2004; Spencer, 2005).

Recent Developments

As noted earlier, retail health clinics are not all the same. Different models have been tried, adopted, modified, and discarded as retailers and their contractors attempt to respond to different market conditions (Dorschner, 2008). Among the most important recent developments are retailers branding their own clinics, retailers co-branding their clinics with others, the movement of health care facilities themselves to offer clinics in retail settings, and the use of telemedicine to connect clinic personnel to clinicians off-site.

Telemedicine is allowing retail health clinics and their personnel to access off-site clinical expertise. Six Houston area Walmart retail clinics operated by My Healthy Access retail clinic company were initially shut down, and then reopened in 2008. These clinics had employed nurse practitioners previously and found that model was not working. The reopened clinics were among the first clinics in the United States to provide services through telemedicine, linking the clinics to local family practice and emergency medicine physicians. They developed a partnership between My Healthy Access and NuPhysicia (Perin, 2008).

While a typical retail clinic is staffed by nurse practitioners on the premises, these clinics are staffed by on-site paramedics who are linked to community physicians via video technology. The paramedics serve as the doctor's "hands," checking vital signs and examining physical attributes with the on-duty physician watching on a video link. The physician then directs the on-site clinicians as they treat the patient. Unlike the replacement of physicians by nurse practitioners, this is like having the doctor in the room. The doctors are mid- or late-career physicians who are highly experienced in family medicine or emergency medicine (Perin, 2008).

In 2008 Walmart opened its first co-branded retail clinics, which provide another possible model for the future. These clinics are co-branded "The Clinic at Walmart" and are affiliated with local hospitals, which provide the actual service using their employees. The advantage for Walmart is that their customers in various cities may have already visited and be familiar with these hospitals. These clinics represent an initial approach toward a goal of 400 clinics by December 2010. Walmart has stated that it is committed to providing health services that are both accessible and affordable. They would like "The Clinic at Walmart" to be associated with high clinical quality at reasonable prices provided by well-known, local health care institutions. Affordable prices are particularly important since data show that approximately 55 percent of its clinic patients have no insurance.

The company is currently implementing a number of initiatives and services that it believes will enhance access, efficiency, and effectiveness in health service delivery:

- Primary care services for common ailments including ear, nose, and throat conditions.
- Preventive services such as physical exams, inoculations, diagnostic procedures, and health screenings.
- Reduced paperwork due to standardized electronic medical records.
- Patient care delivered by non-physician providers who are able to diagnose, treat, and prescribe as appropriate.

"The Clinic at Walmart" is now owned and operated by St. Vincent Health System in Little Rock, Arkansas. Walmart has also contracted with Houston-based retail clinic operator Redi-Clinic to open in-store clinics at 200 Walmart Supercenters. Walmart also opened a partnership between RediClinic and a Dallas hospital system in 2008 (Robeznieks, 2008). Around the country, hospitals are now affiliated with more than 25 Walmart clinics (Freudenheim, 2009).

The Cleveland Clinic has lent its name and backup services to a string of CVS drugstore clinics in Northeastern Ohio. The Mayo Clinic is also operating one Express Care clinic at a supermarket in Rochester, Minnesota, and a second one across town in a shopping mall. The Mayo Clinic says it opened its clinics after hearing employees and patients say they wanted more convenient treatment for minor medical problems (Freudenheim, 2009).

Responsiveness to Top Ten Consumer Hassles

In the previous chapter we identified the top ten consumer hassles that were driving consumers to look for more accessible, more convenient, and less expensive alternatives to traditional health care providers, especially for basic health care needs. In this section we will identify whether and to what degree retail clinics might be able to address or alleviate each of these hassles.

The first hassle was problems in getting appointments. Obviously, retail clinics are one approach for relieving this problem since no appointments are necessary at retail clinics. The second hassle was long waits for services. While long waits could conceivably occur at a particular clinic at a particular time, such waits are not common. Patients are usually seen soon after they arrive.

The third hassle was the small amount of time patients spend with physicians. Retail clinics typically do not employ physicians, although telemedicine might change that dynamic as off-site physicians guide on-site clinicians in their diagnosis and treatment. Surveys of patient satisfaction in retail clinics indicate that service providers do spend sufficient time so that the patients do not feel rushed.

The fourth consumer hassle was administrative paperwork. Other than the medical record routinely maintained by most retail clinics, there is no paperwork required by the clinics other than registration and insurance status. Patient paperwork is minimal. The fifth hassle was inadequate parking or easy access. Since retail stores rely on adequate parking for drivers, geographic and parking access is typically adequate.

The sixth hassle was geographic inconvenience of centralized facilities. Obviously retail clinics are closer to where people live and therefore more accessible. As they grow in numbers, this accessibility should continue to increase. The seventh consumer hassle was inconvenient service hours particularly at night and on weekends. Obviously retail clinics offer extensive weekend and evening hours when other offices may not be available.

The eighth hassle was the escalating cost of health services including out-of-pocket costs. Retail clinics typically take insurance if consumers have insurance and charge less than emergency departments or physician offices for the same services. Consequently, they contribute toward cost containment for consumers. The ninth hassle is communication breakdowns among health care providers. Most retail clinics do have electronic medical records and are ready, willing, and able to communicate to other providers who also have electronic medical records. Thus, retail clinics enhance communication with other providers who are technologically sophisticated, to the benefit of their patients.

The tenth and final hassle is that there is no one-stop shopping so that patients must visit numerous providers to complete their care process. Obviously, retail clinics do not provide the full range of primary, secondary, and tertiary services. Consequently, they cannot be a one-stop shopping site for all services required by all patients. However, they do offer a one-stop shop for those services they do provide, including laboratory services, pharmaceutical services, and electronic medical records. They may also save consumers time by allowing them to shop for other necessities in the same facility where family members may access health services.

CONCLUSIONS AND IMPLICATIONS

Retail clinics have evolved in a time when our health care system is overstressed and not meeting the needs of many Americans. The current system provides many challenges and impediments for consumers that may be addressed by retail health clinics as they develop more accessible, convenient, and lower cost service options for basic health care needs. Retail clinics have identified a need for some type of change, and they are attempting to fill a niche for unmet primary care services by responding to these unmet consumer needs. They recognize that we have developed a high cost, technologically sophisticated, and sometimes impenetrable health care system.

While disruptive innovation in the delivery system is needed across the board, it has occurred in the form of retail health clinics primarily for primary health care services where consumers pay the bill themselves and, to a lesser degree, primary care services subsidized by insurance. Although there is already a strong market demand for the disruptive innovation of retail clinics in providing primary care services, the changes for comparable innovation for more expensive high-tech health services is less positive (Havighurst, 2008).

It is important to note that although retail clinics have grown rapidly since the mid-2000s, they are readily available in certain geographic regions and states, but not readily available in others. As a result, many U.S. citizens do not yet have access to retail clinic services in their immediate locales. However, forecasts indicate that more than 6,000 clinics will be in operation by 2012 (Pulley, 2008).

It should also be noted that clinics have been more complex and costly to operate than many early estimates (Tu & Cohen, 2008). Consequently, new models are developing that allow co-branding with health care providers who are already well-known in their respective markets. As such, these co-branded clinics are better positioned to attract patients and achieve critical mass. Co-branding seems to be the wave of the future (Bagchi, 2008; Goldstein, 2007).

Despite a variety of uncertainties, we believe that retail health clinics will grow and play an important role in our evolving health care system in the future. While they do not constitute a "silver bullet" for addressing all of our health care needs, they can contribute to enhancing access, convenience, and quality for a limited range of primary care services. Through the use of telemedicine, they also offer an opportunity to provide more sophisticated health services in the future, including specialized care.

REFERENCES

Amit, R., & Zott, C. (2001). "Value creation in e-business." *Strategic Management Journal, 22,* 493–520.

Andrews, M. (July 18, 2004). "Next to the express check out, express medical care." *New York Times.* Available at www.nytimes.com.

Armstrong, D. (May 7, 2008). "Health clinics inside stores likely to slow their growth." *Wall Street Journal.*

Bagchi, S. (February 1, 2008). "Mayo Clinic enters retail care business." *Health Care News.* Available at http://www.heartland.org/policybot/results.html?articleid=22571.

Beckham, D. (2002). "Emulating Wal-Mart." *Health Forum Journal, 45*(4), 37–38.

Center for Studying Health System Change. 2007. "Community tracking study household survey." http://www.hschange.com/index.cgi?data=02 (accessed December 1, 2009).

Charitou, C. D., & Markides, C. C. (2003). "Responses to disruptive strategic innovation." *Sloan Management Review, 44*(2), 55–63.

Christensen, C. M., Anthony, S. D., & Roth, E. A. (2004). *Seeing what's next: Using theories of innovation to predict industry change.* Boston: Harvard Business School Press.

Christensen, C. M., Bohmer, R., & Kenagy, J. (2000, September/October). "Will disruptive innovations cure health care?" *Harvard Business Review, 78*(5), 102–111.

Christiansen, C. M., Johnson, M. W., & Dann, J. (2002). "November." Disrupt and Prosper. Optimizemag.com 41–48.

"'The Clinic at Wal-Mart' to Open in Atlanta, Little Rock and Dallas Supercenters." (2008). http://Wal-Martstores.com/FactsNews/NewsRoom/7922.aspx (accessed February 11, 2009).

Convenient Care Association. 2007. "History of the CCI." http://www.convenientcareassociation.org/abouthcci.htm (accessed January 31, 2008).

Cunningham, P. J., & Felland, L. E. (2008). "Falling behinds: American's access to medical care deteriorates 2003–2007." Tracking Report No. 19. Washington, DC: Center for Studying Health System Change.

Day, J. D., & Wendler, J. C. (1998). "The new economics of organization." *The McKinsey Quarterly, 1,* 5–18.

Dorschner, J. (2008). "Walk-in clinics spread as others close down." http://www.miamiherald.com/152/v-print/story/398857.html (accessed January 30, 2009).

Fottler, M. D., & Malvey, D. (2007). "Strategic entrepreneurship in the health care industry: The case of Wal-Mart." In J. D. Blair & M. D. Fottler (Eds.), *Strategic thinking and entrepreneurial action in health care* (pp. 257–278). Amsterdam, Holland: Elsevier/JAI Press.

Freudenheim, M. (2009). "Hospitals begin to move into supermarkets." *The New York Times.* http://nytimes.com/2009/05/12/business/12 clinic.html?pagewanted=print (accessed May 12, 2009).

Goldstein, J. (2007, May 16). "Some health systems out to beat retailers at clinic game." *Wall Street Journal Health Blog.*

Harris Interactive. (April 11, 2007). "Most adults satisfied with care at retail based health clinics." *Health Care Poll, 6*(6).

Havigurst, C. C. (2008). "Disruptive innovation: The demand side." *Health Affairs, 27*(5), 1341–1344.

Hitt, M. A., & Ireland, R. D. (2000). "The intersection of entrepreneurship and strategic management research." In D. L. Sexton and H. Landstrom (Eds.), *Handbook of Entrepreneurship* (pp. 45–63). Oxford: Blackwell Publishers.

Hitt, M. A., Ireland, R. D., Camp, S. M., & Sexton, D. L. (2001). "Strategic entrepreneurship: Entrepreneurship strategies for wealth creation." *Strategic Management Journal, 22,* 479–491.

Ireland, R. D., Hitt, M. A., & Sirmon, D. G. (2003). "A model of strategic entrepreneurship: The construct and its dimensions." *Journal of Management, 29*(6), 963–989.

Kluge, J., Meffert, J., & Stein, L. (2000). "The German road to innovation." *The McKinsey Quarterly, 2,* 99–105.

Lin, D. Q. (2008). "Convenience care clinics: Opposition, opportunity, and the path to health system integration." *Frontiers of Health Services Management, 24*(3), 3–11.

Malvey, D., & Fottler, M. D. (2006). "The retail revolution in health care: Who will win and who will lose?" *Health Care Management Review, 31*(3), 168–178.

Mehrotra, A., Wang, M. C., Lave, J. R., Adams, J. L., & McGlynn, E. A. (2008). "Retail clinics, primary care physicians, and emergency departments: A comparison of physician business." *Health Affairs, 27*(5), 1275–1282.

Perin, M. (August 6, 2008). "Retail health clinics reopen with new model." *Houston Business Journal.* http://houston.bizjournals.com/houston/stories/2008/08/04 (accessed February 3, 2009).

"PRN and the Cleveland Clinic team up to provide health tips on the Wal-Mart TV Network." (June 20, 2005). Retrieved July 28, 2005, from http://www.mywire.com/a/PRNewswire/PRN-Cleveland-Clinic-Team-Up/901675/.

Pollert, P., Dobberstein, D., & Wiisanen, R. (2008). "Jumping into the health care retail market: Our experience." *Frontiers of Health Services Management, 24*(3), 13–21.

PricewaterhouseCoopers. (2005). *Management Barometer Survey.* New York: PricewaterhouseCoopers.

Pulley, J. (April 28, 2008). "Store-based clinics face rocky regulatory landscape." *Government Health IT.* http://www.govhealthit.com/online/news/350330-1.html.

Rice, B. (September 16, 2005). "In-store clinics: Should you worry?" *Medical Economics.* Retrieved December 31, 2005, from http://www.memag.com/memag/article/articleDetail.jsp?id=179078&sk=&date=&&pageID=1.

Robeznieks, A. (2008). "Wal-Mart opening co-branded store in clinics." ModernHealthcare.com (accessed February 7, 2008).

Schoonhoven, C. B., & Romanelli, E. (2001). "Emergent themes and the next wave of entrepreneurial research." In C. B. Schoonhoven & E. Romanelli (Eds.), *The entrepreneurship dynamic: Origins of entrepreneurship and the evaluation of industries* (pp. 383–408). Stanford, CA: Stanford University Press.

Schumpeter, J. A. (1934). *The theory of economic development.* Cambridge, MA: Harvard University Press.

Scott, M. K. (2006, July). *Healthcare in the express lane: The emergence of retail clinics.* Report to the California Healthcare Foundation.

Scott, M. K. (2008). Interview with Mary Kate Scott, conducted July 2008, cited in Tu and Cohen, 2008.

Spencer, J. (October 5, 2005). "Getting your healthcare at Wal-Mart." *Wall Street Journal, 266*(70), D1, D5.

Starr, P. (1982). *The social transformation of American medicine.* New York: Basic Books, Inc.

Tu, H. T., & Cohen, G. R. (2008, December). "Checking up on retail based health clinics: Is the boom ending?" *The Commonwealth Fund.* Issues Brief No. 1199. New York: The Commonwealth Fund.

Tushman, M. L., & O'Reilly, C. A. (1996). "Ambidextrous organizations: Managing evolutionary and revolutionary change." *California Management Review, 38*(4), 8–30.

Chapter 5

The Retail Clinic

OVERVIEW

Health care is a business. In the nineteenth and early twentieth centuries, doctors bartered their services, often accepting farm products or crafts from patients in exchange for treatment. The transaction between the patient and provider was arm's length. But all of that changed with the introduction of health insurance in the mid-twentieth century. Increasingly, third-party payers (i.e., government, insurers, and employers) assumed control of the pricing and purchasing of health care (Starr, 1982). Providing health care services became more of a *wholesale* business with doctors and hospitals selling their services to third-party payers instead of directly to patients (Honaman, 2006, p. 49).

However, the emergence of the retail clinic offers consumers an alternative to wholesale health care. Retail involves selling small quantities of goods and services directly to the consumer. Consequently, there is no middleman (third-party payer) so the costs are reduced.

Retail clinics, also known as retail-based health clinics or convenient care clinics, have become one of the fastest growing segments of the health care sector (Costello, 2008). Even though thousands of freestanding primary care clinics have been operating across the United States, including many in shopping mall locations, they have been staffed primarily by physicians. The retail health clinics represent a new model for primary care services for the consumer. They offer a limited number of services at lower prices and almost always are staffed by a nurse practitioner (Turner, 2007).

Despite rapid growth and increasing national attention to retail clinics, these clinics are still a fairly new phenomenon, and little is known about them. There are few sources of reliable information and studies that detail and describe these clinics. However, what has been suggested by consumers and researchers alike is that retail clinics represent an affordable alternative for primary care. They offer increased access to groups that typically have difficulty accessing health care services, especially the uninsured and minorities. Yet, as of 2007 only 2.3 percent of families in the United States reported ever having visited a retail clinic (Tu & Cohen, 2008).

At the beginning of 2006, there were only 60 retail clinics in the United States (Consumer Reports, 2009, April). By the end of 2008, industry experts Merchant Medicine reported a year of record growth for retail clinics. There were approximately 1,175 retail clinics located in 37 different states, with Florida reporting the highest number of retail clinics in operation (122) than any other state. This represents a net increase of 274 clinics from 2007. In addition, a total of 55 retail clinic operators were identified, and 43 different retailers were reported as "hosting" these clinics in their stores. In the host capacity, the retailer functions as a landlord and leases space to the clinic operator (Merchant Medicine, 2009e).

In the face of such positive growth, however, there was a more significant development: clinic closures. Approximately 150 retail clinics were closed during 2008, and about 80 of the closures were the result of some privately backed clinic operators going out of business while others exited because they were not willing to wait up to two years for profits (Merchant Medicine, 2009e).

In addition, the retailers associated with retail clinics began to change their strategies. Some retail pharmacy chains began pursuing acquisition strategies and buying clinic operators. Meanwhile the world's largest discount retailer, Walmart, has rejected buying clinic operators and prefers to function as a landlord. However, Walmart continues to experiment and test different clinic models, including a telemedicine model, as well as partnering with hospital system owned clinics in an effort to co-brand the retail clinic.

This chapter seeks to answer the following five questions and provide some insight into retail clinics and their potential to change the delivery of health care services:

1. What do we know about retail clinics?
2. What is the business model and strategy of retail clinics?

   - Who are the owners of retail clinics?
   - What role has retail giant Walmart played?

3. What are the barriers and facilitators of their growth and expansion?

- Can they survive the regulatory environment?
- Are they profitable?
- Do they satisfy consumer needs for quality of care?

4. How do retail clinics "fit" with health care reform efforts?
5. What does the future predict for retail clinics?

WHAT DO WE KNOW ABOUT RETAIL CLINICS?

Retail clinics are in many ways an experiment that links retailers and health care (Scott, 2006). Clinics are typically located in retail stores such as Walmart, Target, Walgreens, and CVS, and grocery chains such as Publix or Kroger. Therefore, instead of the consumer entering the health care system in the routine manner by visiting a physician in his office or the emergency room, patients may now access health care when they go shopping. This means that there is a new portal of entry to the health care system for the consumer, one that lies outside of *mainstream* health care (Tu & Cohen, 2008).

By offering patients a new portal for medical care, retailers are separating basic health care services from traditional providers and offering patients a means of escaping what has previously been a captive system. This captive system has contained few alternatives for patients, especially within the restrictions of tightly managed medical care. Retailers are also revising the relationship with the patient's physician who is not involved in the decision to seek services at a retail health care clinic. Such changes will require a new logic about marketing as customers toggle between retail and traditional health care system boundaries.

Birth of the Retail Clinic

The retail clinic was born in 2000 in the Minneapolis–St. Paul metropolitan area. The first clinic operator, a private, for-profit group, was founded by Rick Krieger, whose business model was based on his personal experience in spending hours trying to get his son an appointment to see a doctor for a strep throat test. Krieger's idea was simple: It should not take two hours waiting in a clinic or an emergency department to obtain a simple diagnostic test. Krieger and his business partners subsequently developed a retail clinic model that was operated by a company called Quick-Medx, which later became MinuteClinic (Scott, 2006).

Even though retail clinics have expanded across the United States, the Minneapolis–St. Paul metropolitan area continues to claim the largest number of clinics, 61 (Merchant Medicine, 2009f). The area also ranks number one for high use: 191,000 families reported having used retail clinics in 2008. This represents 6.4 percent of the state population (Tu & Cohen, 2008).

In a report prepared for the California HealthCare Foundation, Mary Kate Scott offered the following definition of a retail clinic that distinguishes it from other types of clinics:

> A medical clinic located within a larger retail operation that offers general medical services (as opposed to specialty clinics such as eye care) to the public on an ongoing (rather than one-time or seasonal) basis. These clinics differ from both urgent care clinics or the "Doc in a box" concept in several ways: a limited service offering (increasing speed), a co-location with pharmacy (increasing convenience), and lower cost structure (reducing prices). (Scott, 2006, p. 9)

Retail clinics are not freestanding. They are located within a retail establishment. The clinics occupy a small amount of space within the retail establishment, usually about 200–500 square feet. The setup is also minimal with a reception desk and one or two exam rooms (Scott, 2006, p. 9).

Retail clinics offer quick access to common or basic health care services for such illnesses as earaches and sore throats, as well as for providing immunizations and preventive screenings. They are staffed by nurse practitioners, physician assistants, or advanced practice nurses who can legally treat patients and write prescriptions in most states. Physician backup is usually available through telephone or email (Spencer, 2005).

New Portal of Care

Retail clinics function as a *portal* to the primary care system, especially for those who do not have a regular source of care. In the Rand Corporation Study (2008), which analyzed data for 1.3 million clinic visits from 2000 through 2007, fully 60 percent of those surveyed did not have a primary care physician (PCP). Young adults (ages 18–44) in particular did not have a regular source of care, and they accounted for 43 percent of all clinic visits (Mehrotra et al., 2008).

Most of the users of retail clinics appear to understand that retail clinic visits are for basic medical needs, including minor injuries and illnesses. Only 2.3 percent of clinic patients end up being referred to the emergency department. Listed below are the ten simple conditions and preventive care that were identified in the Rand Corporation Study as reasons for visiting a retail clinic. They represented approximately 90 percent of retail clinic visits:

1. Upper respiratory infections
2. Sinusitis
3. Bronchitis
4. Sore throat
5. Immunizations
6. Inner ear infections
7. Swimmer's ear
8. Conjunctivitis
9. Urinary tract infections
10. And either a screening test or a blood test (Mehrotra et al., 2008).

Meanwhile, another major study looked at family use of retail clinics. The researchers analyzed data from the 2007 Health Tracking Household Survey that was conducted by the Center for Studying Health System Change. The analysis revealed that users tended to be younger families and people who had difficulty gaining access to the health care system, including the uninsured and minorities. Uninsured families accounted for 27 percent of retail clinic visits. The finding that such families used clinics at a much higher rate than their share of the population is consistent with previous research about uninsured consumers (Tu & Cohen, 2008, pp. 3–4).

Most clinics offer extended hours, including evening hours and weekends. Typically no appointments are needed, and there is little waiting time. Clinic visits tend to be brief or about 15 minutes. Patients usually can use waiting time productively by shopping elsewhere in the store (Andrews, 2004; Rice, 2005; Spencer, 2005). The charges for services at a retail clinic tend to be much lower than what would be expected in an emergency department or physician practice.

Health care innovations precipitated the development of retail clinics. Retail clinics are possible because of cost-reducing innovations in health care such as the development of inexpensive yet reliable tests for strep throat and other infections. They are also possible because of the development of rules-based treatment protocols that expand diagnostic and treatment capabilities of non-physician providers such as nurse practitioners (Robinson & Smith, 2008).

WHAT IS THE BUSINESS MODEL AND STRATEGY OF RETAIL CLINICS?

The business model of the retail clinic is pretty straightforward. The value proposition for retail clinics includes quick, inexpensive, and convenient care. Both the business and operational models are dependent on a limited services menu, similar to the fast food industry. The listed services are highly standardized interventions such as vaccinations and tests and treatments for bronchitis and ear infections that require no physician evaluation. In addition, the clinics are affiliated with drugstores, which facilitates the filling of prescriptions on the spot (Bohmer, 2007, p. 766).

Common elements of the business model include:

- Location in a retail store
- Use of electronic medical records
- Use of electronic standardized diagnostic and treatment protocols
- Care by a nurse practitioner
- Limited range of services
- No appointment necessary
- Affiliation with a pharmacy
- Extended hours (i.e., nights and weekends)

One of the primary means of making health care better and less expensive involves generating new business models. Even though the business model for the retail clinic is fairly simple, it nevertheless reflects innovation in service delivery because it is a consumer-focused model (Herzlinger, 2006, pp. 63–65). It also concentrates on basic health care services, which are low end or less expensive to provide. The model's innovation also centers on giving the consumer value and convenience (Deloitte, 2008).

Changing from a Cash-Based to Insurance Coverage

In the early years, most clinics initially operated as a strictly "cash-based" business (Woznicki, 2004). However, a major development has been the move to secure insurance coverage for clinic visits (Laws & Scott, 2008). The Rand Corporation study found that two-thirds of their large sample of retail clinic visits were paid for with insurance (Mehrotra et al., 2008). Humana, UnitedHealth Group, Aetna, and Cigna cover retail clinic visits (Associated Press, 2007).

For example, Cigna covers care at a variety of retail clinic outlets including MinuteClinic, RediClinic, Take Care Health System, Little Clinic, as well as Cigna Medical Group (CMG) Care Today Clinics, which are freestanding clinics with extended hours. Furthermore, they are covering such visits much the way they would cover a visit to the primary care physician. Cigna processes retail clinic claims at the same benefit level as an office visit to a primary care physician (Bazzoli, 2008). Blue Cross Blue Shield of Minnesota reported reducing or waiving co-payments for a number of member companies who use MinuteClinics and several other store-based clinics (Associated Press, 2007).

By 2007 all major national private insurance carriers had begun covering retail clinic visits and also working with clinic operators to expedite claims processing (Scott, 2007; Tu & Cohen, 2008). Meanwhile, in 2007 several large clinic operators, including MinuteClinic and RediClinic met both federal and state requirements to receive reimbursement for public insurance programs Medicare and Medicaid (Tu & Cohen, 2008). An exception to the trend toward attaining insurance coverage is California-based QuickHealth, a physician-staffed model that has refused to seek insurance reimbursement (Laws & Scott, 2008).

WHO ARE THE OWNERS OF RETAIL CLINICS?

In the early years, 2000–2006, the clinics typically were not owned, staffed, or managed by retailers. The clinics were owned by privately backed companies. Retailers viewed the clinics as a means to capture the loyalty of consumers for broader commercial purposes (Winkenwerder, 2008). The retailer functioned as a host. As subcontractors, clinic owners usually were entirely responsible for clinic operations, including liability insurance (Spencer, 2005). Meanwhile, retailers set the terms for such elements and in-store advertising and marketing. Initially, many retail clinic operators were desperate to set up shop in busy retail stores and they negotiated poor terms. The retailer has a one-time cost of about $20,000 to $100,000 to make the space ready for the clinic company. The clinic company pays to physically retrofit the space to its needs. The average setup cost is about $50,000, a sizable investment for the clinic company (Scott, 2006, p. 9).

However, unlike the health care industry, retail products have limited life cycles and retailers constantly revise their formats and services to eliminate less profitable lines of business (Scott, 2006). The retail mentality of "fast turnaround, rapid consumer testing, and constant reinvention of the model" (Scott, 2006, p. 10) is rare in health care. This means that the retail clinic model will continue to evolve.

Thus, ownership of the in-store clinics will shift. Physician entrepreneurs have developed some clinics. Other clinics are owned or capitalized by equity investment firms. For example, Revolution Health Group recently established by AOL co-founder Steve Case has capitalized RediClinics. These are retail-based health clinics, which are located inside popular retail outlets such as Walmart stores (PRN Newswire, 2005).

Perhaps the most significant changes in the model and strategy have been the trend toward ownership of retail clinics by large pharmacy chains and the growth of hospital-linked retail clinics. In 2009, retail clinic ownership fell into three categories described below and further elaborated on in Table 5.1.

1. Retail pharmacy-owned clinics, which represents the largest number of clinics
2. Privately backed clinic operators representing investors and entrepreneurs
3. Hospital-linked retail clinic operators.

TABLE 5.1   Top Retail Clinic Operators by Type and Number

Clinic Operator	Type	Number
MinuteClinic (CVS)	Retail pharmacy owned	550
Take Care (Walgreens)	Retail pharmacy owned	318
The Little Clinic (Kroger)	Retail pharmacy owned	91
Target Clinic (Target)	Retail pharmacy owned	28
RediClinic (Revolution Health/Steve Case)	Privately backed (investors/entrepreneurs)	21
Aurora QuickCare	Hospital system owned	19

Source: Merchant Medicine 2008 year end Review and 2009 Outlook.

The Trend Toward Retail Pharmacy-Owned Clinics

The trend has been toward retailers acquiring ownership of the clinic company at least with pharmacy retailers and grocery chains. The majority of clinics are owned by large retail pharmacy chains (987). This change revises the retail clinic model, giving the retailer more control over the clinic and the opportunity to create downstream business from the clinic. For example, retail clinics can add to their prescription counter business, which has been estimated as high as 70 percent of their revenue (Merchant Medicine, 2009d).

In addition, even though retail-based pharmacy clinics are not making money in some markets, they can afford to finance their own expansions. For example, Walgreens expects it to take up to two years for a retail clinic to make a profit. It purchased Take Care Health Systems in 2007 and is reportedly financing its own clinic expansions (Japsen, 2008).

In 2006 MinuteClinics was purchased by CVS, the retail pharmacy chain. Together MinuteClinics and Take Care Health represent 74 percent of the retail clinics open in the United States. MinuteClinics operates the largest number of clinics, 550, as reported in December 2008 (Merchant Medicine, 2009d). Its closest competitor, Walgreen's Take Care Health reported a total of 334 retail clinics for 2008 (Merchant Medicine, 2009a) and is the leader in opening new clinics. Take Care Health added 187 clinics in 2008 compared with MinuteClinics adding only 92 new clinics (Merchant Medicine, 2009d).

In addition, Take Care Health acquired two of the largest operators of on-site employer clinics, Whole Health and CHD Meridian, both of which were subsumed under a new operating division called Health and Wellness. Walgreens has begun to market a combination of its clinics, pharmacies, and other services to businesses looking to save on employee health care costs. MinuteClinics does not have the on-site employer clinic capabilities of Take Care Health. However, both entities are engaged in pharmacy benefits management programs for self-insured employers (Merchant Medicine, 2009d).

Target Clinic is also included under pharmacy-owned retailers because its pharmacy division runs the retail clinic operation. Before August 2008, these clinics were operated by Medcor, which is best known for its operation of on-site clinics for a variety of large companies including other retailers and some hospital systems. At this time (2009) there are no immediate plans for Target to grow their retail clinics (Merchant Medicine, 2009d). The Little Clinic is a retail clinic company that previously was supported by venture capitalists (Solera) and has seen significant investment by the large retail grocer Kroger, which also has in-store pharmacy service.

Privately Backed Clinic Operators: Investors and Entrepreneurs

It was reported that there were only 10 privately backed retail clinic operators, representing a total of 67 retail clinics as of 2008 (Merchant Medicine, 2009d). Many of the retail clinic companies have dropped out. Those that remain have been financed by formidable competing entrepreneurs, including Stephen M. Case, the former AOL chairman and founder of Revolution Health, and Richard L. Scott, who once ran the nation's largest for-profit hospital chain, Columbia/HCA (Freudenheim, 2006). Case is associated with RediClinics and Scott with Solantic.

Rediclinics owns about 21 clinics. They subcontract with retailers such as Walmart, but also enter into partnerships with hospital systems. As a rule, RediClinics tends to partner with the largest hospital in each city in which it locates. This is so doctors there can consult with the clinic (Basler, 2007). Meanwhile, Solantic is based in Jacksonville, Florida, and differs from the typical retail clinic in that its clinics are staffed by doctors and provide a wide range of services. Many of the routine services may be slightly higher priced than at other competitors (Freudenheim, 2006). Solantic was founded in 2001 and opened its first clinic in a Walmart (Fineman, 2006). Solantic is privately funded, including a $100 million investment in 2007 by New York City–based private equity firm Welsh, Carson, Anderson, and Stone (Bowling, 2007).

A new retail clinic venture plans to focus on airport locations, beginning in Georgia. The venture, AeroClinic, launched its first clinic at the main terminal of one of the world's busiest airports, Atlanta's Hartsfield-Jackson Airport. AeroClinic's founders include former U.S. Surgeon General Dr. David Satcher, who also serves on the company's board of directors. The clinic will offer routine care for minor ailments, but will also offer preventive testing, physical exams, and routine immunizations. The clinic accepts Aetna coverage. The company expects to expand into the community retail business under a brand called AmeriClinic

(FierceHealthcare, 2007a). Even though pharmacies and clinics are common in foreign airports, they are a new market for retail clinics. Other companies that expect to open clinics at airports are Solantic and AirportMD (FierceHealthcare, 2008a).

Hospital-linked Retail Clinics

Even though retailer-owned clinics are the predominant business model, there is growth in the market involving hospital and health system ownership of clinics. This development bears watching according to Mary Kate Scott, industry expert (Porter, 2008). Hospital-linked retail clinics may become the predominant model. At least one in ten retail clinics has a connection with a hospital (Fruedeheim, 2009).

Hospital systems have emerged as key "players" among retail clinics. Hospital systems have two reasons to adopt the retail clinic model. First, the clinics represent a source of new patients for both the hospital and physicians. They also are expected to increase "downstream" revenue with follow-up care and ancillary services (Litch, 2008). More importantly, they represent a defensive strategy to protect their "turf" from competitors (Newbold & O'Neil, 2008, p. 25).

The sentiment against retail clinics remains strong among physicians, but hospital systems appear to be changing strategies. Instead of competing directly with these clinics, they have partnered with them. In 2009, there are reportedly 30 hospital systems that operate 108 retail clinics across the United States (Merchant Medicine, 2009e). This strategy reflects a key stakeholder management principle that advocates turning competitors into collaborators. Thus, the success of a competitor, i.e., the retail clinic, in turn becomes the success of the hospital system.

For example, in 2009 MinuteClinics announced collaboration with the prestigious Cleveland Clinic, a collaboration that will include nine locations in northeast Ohio. The Cleveland Clinic will provide clinical consultations to the nurse practitioners that staff each clinic (Immediate Care Business, 2009). In addition, the Mayo Clinic will open retail clinics through *Mayo Express Care* (Kaisernetwork, 2007c). These collaborative partnerships permit the retailer to co-brand with a prestigious hospital or health care system while simultaneously providing the system access to an extensive population of patients.

Partnering with a Privately Backed Clinic Operator

Memorial Hermann Healthcare System in Houston, Texas, is an example of a hospital system that has partnered with a privately backed company, RediClinic. In early 2007, Hermann created a "joint venture" partnership with RediClinic. Primary care physicians who are affiliated with the hospital are on-site at the Redi-Clinics approximately 20 percent of the hours that they are open. Memorial Hermann did not have hospitals or urgent care facilities within many of the zip code markets that were being targeted by RediClinic. Therefore, RediClinic access points offered a new source of patient referrals for the hospital and physician offices (Fenn, 2008).

In addition to the RediClinics, the hospital system owns and operates two retail clinics called Neighborcare clinics. These two clinics are strategically located near two Memorial Hermann community hospital emergency departments. If patients are nonemergent and are able to pay cash for their care, they are shifted from the emergency department to the retail clinics, which are staffed by nurse practitioners from the hospital. In this way, both the hospital and the patient avoid a high cost emergency department visit for routine care (Fenn, 2008). In addition, it reduces unnecessary crowding in the emergency department with patients seeking routine care. Finally, it *converts* a nonpaying patient into one who can pay because of more affordable pricing. This would appear to be a win-win situation for hospitals, physicians, and patients.

Memorial Hermann and RediClinics subsequently expanded their relationship, creating a 50/50 joint venture for Houston Redi-Clinics. The new relationship eventually resulted in the creation of a board of directors with equal representation from the hospital system and RediClinics (Fenn, 2008).

Aurora QuickCare is owned by Aurora Health Care, a nonprofit Wisconsin health care system whose goals are aimed at increasing access to health care for its communities (Rice, 2005). The benefits to hospital systems include operating profit and bringing new patients into their systems, especially patients who do not have a primary care physician. Aurora has clinics located in Walmart stores.

WHAT ROLE HAS WALMART PLAYED?

Walmart, the largest retailer in North America and the world, is widely recognized for revolutionizing retailing and creating an intensely competitive retail market. By singularly focusing on its customers; satisfying them through value and low prices, Walmart has transformed the retail industry and set its standards (Bergdahl, 2004). However, with the advent of relatively flat sales, Walmart and other large retailers have been examining new markets, including health care.

Within the past few years, these retailers have introduced a variety of health care products and services, including in-store health clinics. They have also revised their operating structure and hired people with broad-based expertise in health care. For example, in 2007 Walmart announced that it had hired Dr. John Agwunobi, who at the time was the current assistant secretary for the U.S. Department of Health and Human Services and is also a public health expert. Dr. Agwunobi was hired as senior vice president and president for Professional Services Division in the United States. His responsibilities include overseeing the company's health and wellness business, including health care clinics (Walmart Stores, 2009).

Walmart, the world's largest retailer, continues to adhere to the original "host" model for retail clinics. Walmart continues to lease space in its stores rather than purchase clinic operators as the retail pharmacy chains have done. One reason for doing so may be that retail clinics present the potential for significant medical liability cases. Trial attorneys can be expected to find that the "deep pockets" of large corporations such as Walmart are far more attractive than that of a physician (Winkenwerder, 2008).

Walmart also continues to test different clinic models, including a telemedicine model that uses physicians, paramedics, and video link technology. The physician on duty will watch the patient through the video link and direct paramedics to conduct treatments (Perin, 2008). Walmart is also moving into new markets such as electronic health records for physician practices (Lohr, 2009).

In addition, Walmart has also made a major departure from its existing pattern with retail clinics. Walmart is pursuing a co-branding strategy that uses clinics that are owned and operated by local health systems and hospitals. Walmart has dramatically decreased the number of clinics backed by private investors and has begun replacing them with hospital system operators that perform under a co-branding arrangement (Merchant Medicine, 2009d). Integrating with an existing health system confers a sense of legitimacy and reputation on the clinic such that people who visit a Walmart can identify the brand of care with the hospital system.

Walmart opened its first in-store medical clinic under its own name, *The Clinic at Walmart*, in April 2008 as a joint venture with several local hospital and health systems in Dallas, Atlanta, and Little Rock, Arkansas. This appears to be part of a larger strategy in which Walmart is seeking collaboration with local health care providers to build trust among local shoppers (FierceHealthcare, 2008f; Associated Press, 2008). On the Walmart Web site, the following statement is posted regarding The Clinic at Walmart:

> "The Clinic at Walmart": A direct link between the community and local hospitals. Over the next two years, we intend to partner with local hospitals to open "The Clinic at Walmart" co-branded clinics in our stores. These co-branded clinics will be directly linked to the hospitals our customers already know and trust. Each clinic will offer a set of affordable "Get Well" and "Stay Well" services designed to treat common ailments and other preventative care. (Walmart Stores, 2009)

As retailers move into health care markets, they look to enhance image and reputation through linkages with other key health care stakeholders. Walmart has looked to other outlets to achieve brand identity for its health care products and lines. For example, Walmart has earlier partnered with the Cleveland Clinic, which is consistently named one of the nation's best hospitals by *U.S. News and World Report*, to provide health information to viewers of the Walmart Television Network. This includes Pharmacy TV that is located within Walmart pharmacies (PRN Newswire, 2005).

Walmart also partnered with Humana, Inc., one of the largest health benefits companies in the United States, to offer a Medicare prescription drug card featuring both the Humana and Walmart brands. This linkage is part of an aggressive marketing campaign by Humana to increase its Medicare business and expand its coverage from 25 to 46 states within the next year (Schreiner, 2005).

Walmart has also tested other care services, including treatments to relieve back pain. Back pain is the eighth-leading reason for doctor visits, and approximately 65 million people in the United States are affected by it. Roughly $26 million is spent annually to treat back pain. The uninsured are particular targets for such services because of the low cost and the option of purchasing one treatment at a time. Walmart has a lease agreement with America's

Back, a for-profit company that provides in-store back pain clinics in various Colorado store locations (Alsever, 2004).

Revamping the Market for Prescription Drugs

In 2006, Walmart changed the way prescriptions are priced for both consumers and employers. They did so first for consumers by offering hundreds of generic prescriptions at the cost of $4 per prescription. Even though there is no estimate of actual sales volume that shifted to Walmart as a result of this change, customers have saved $800 million in prescription costs. Competitors such as Walgreens and CVS have subsequently matched Walmart's pricing (Newbold & O'Neil, 2008).

Walmart has also aimed its strategy for lower prescription drug prices directly at employers. In 2008, Walmart test piloted a program with Caterpillar, Inc., to streamline the way drugs are purchased and priced. Walmart contracts with Caterpillar to waive the $5 co-payment for Caterpillar employees on any generic drugs if they purchase them at a Walmart Pharmacy or Sam's Club Pharmacy. Caterpillar has about 70,000 employees and retirees using the Walmart program (Jones, 2009).

Walmart's new program is very different from the way most employers purchase drugs, which is through a middleman or pharmacy benefit manager. Walmart's program eliminates the middleman and the ability to inflate prices. The price Walmart charges Caterpillar for drugs is based on the price it paid the drug manufacturer, plus a markup for overhead and profit. The results of the test efforts were successful, and Walmart is exploring implementing programs with other firms. Meanwhile Walgreens reports that they are pursuing a similar strategy with employers, but intend to have a more comprehensive offering that combines lower drug prices, health and wellness clinics, and retail clinics located at corporation sites (Jones, 2009).

WHAT ARE THE BARRIERS AND FACILITATORS TO THE GROWTH AND EXPANSION OF RETAIL CLINICS?

Medical Community

In the beginning, the medical community closely scrutinized the growth of retail clinics. Some physicians pointed to the existence of retail clinics as more evidence of the country's deteriorating system of health care, especially a failing primary care infrastructure (Gammon, 2007). Organizations such as the American Medical Association (AMA), the American Academy of Pediatrics (AAP), and the American Academy of Family Physicians (AAFP) have called for more regulation of these clinics, especially federal laws that would slow the growth of clinics (Japsen, 2007). The AMA also requested the establishment of treatment codes to ensure that these clinics only treated minor maladies and a ban on the practice by which health insurers offer to waive or reduce co-payments for patients who seek care at retail clinics (Kaisernetwork, 2007d; 2007a; 2007b).

In 2007, the president of the AAP, Jay Berkelhamer, issued a position that retail clinics were not appropriate for infants, children, and adolescents. Problems with continuity of care and lack of access to their complete medical history were cited. However, the AMA essentially stepped back from a similar proposal that sought to impose age limits for patients treated at retail clinics (Kaisernetwork, 2007a).

Meanwhile, the AAFP took a proactive stance toward retail clinics, recognizing them for the potential to complement the work of family and other primary care physicians. The AAFP developed a list of guidelines (Desired Attributes of Retail health Clinics) to optimize the care delivered at retail clinics and ensure the scope of practice was adhered to (Denning, 2006). Clinic operators such as Take Care Health Systems initially committed to these guidelines. However, in 2008, Take Care Health Systems informed the AAFP that it would not renew their commitment. Such action fueled speculation that retail clinics might be looking to advance beyond their existing scope of practice, the treatment of simple health problems (Porter, 2008).

Regulatory Environment

One of the biggest challenges to retail clinics may be attempts to regulate clinics to the point where they are not economically viable (Winkenwerder, 2008). The health care sector is covered by regulations that prescribe and proscribe what can be done and who can do it. Some regulations are well intended to protect patients and ensure high quality of care. Yet other regulations are attempts to limit competition, as well as inhibit transparency of pricing and performance information (Robinson & Smith, 2008).

Because health care is largely regulated and licensed at the state level, some states are more receptive to having non-physicians deliver care than others (Turner, 2007). CVS's home is in the state of Rhode Island, but Rhode Island refused to let CVS open retail clinics in the state. Florida operates more clinics than any other state, but requires clinics to post notice whether a physician is present and to also disclose the credentials of clinic staff. California requires the retail clinic to be owned by a physician. Conversely, states such as Texas and Wyoming have reduced the restrictions on clinics, including the types of treatments that nurse practitioners can perform (Kaisernetwork, 2007g; Japsen, 2007b). The Federal Trade Commission has not been supportive of legislative attempts in Illinois to limit the growth of retail clinic industry, especially provisions that would exempt retail clinics from regulation if they were owned by hospitals and physicians (FierceHealthcare, 2008b).

Nowhere is the impact of regulation better observed than in the state of Massachusetts where CVS proposed opening its Minute-Clinics as the state's first retail clinics. CVS attempted to get permission to open its clinics in locations across the Boston metro area. What ensued was a highly visible and protracted battle that included state regulators and Boston Mayor Thomas Menino, who openly opposed the retail clinic model (FierceHealthcare, 2008c; Smith, 2008b).

During hearings held in 2007, the state's Public Health Council considered health regulators' concerns about patients receiving adequate care at retail clinics (Kaisernetwork, 2007g). In January 2008, the Council voted to approve a proposal to permit pharmacies and other retail outlets to open medical clinics in their stores. New rules require the clinics to provide patients and their primary care physicians with access to electronic records of the patients' visits and treatments. Oversight of clinics has been assigned to the state's public health department medical director (Modern Healthcare, 2008; Smith, 2008a).

Despite the opposition to retail clinics in Massachusetts, they appear poised to expand in the state. MinuteClinics is exploring the potential for accessing reimbursement for treating low-income Medicaid patients (Kowalczyk, 2009). In addition, Walgreens asked for permission to open its Take Care Health clinics across the state, thereby putting it in competition with CVS MinuteClinics. Walgreens is looking to Massachusetts for expansion because of the state's move toward almost complete universal health coverage.

Walgreens expects its retail clinics to provide more access points to get patients into the system as well as meet the demands of the growing shortage of primary care practitioners in the state (Smith, 2008b; Smith, 2008c).

Are They Profitable?

Currently there is little evidence to demonstrate how retail clinics will fare long term, and privately held companies do not have to release financial details. However, start-up costs are high, about $50,000, and even though nurse practitioners are less expensive to employ than physicians, their salaries range between $65,000 and $80,000 compared with physicians whose salaries are up to twice that amount.

It has been estimated that retail clinics must see between 17 and 23 patients a day to stay in business. In 2006, the average Minute-Clinic reported seeing 25–30 patients a day. Fifty to sixty percent of these visitors turned out to be new pharmacy customers. And 53 percent of patients who visit a MinuteClinic go on to buy other merchandise at the store within which they are located (Ramachandran, 2006; Scott, 2006).

Heavy patient volumes are essential in these clinics, and clinic operators must wait anywhere from 18 months to two years to reach the breakeven point. Annualized operating expenses are expected to be in excess of $250,000 for the "average" retail clinic. The total amount of capital, including excess capital to achieve breakeven, is estimated to be in the $600,000 to $700,000 range. Few clinics can be expected to generate sufficient patient revenue in these clinics to offset the operating expenses in the early stages (Newbold & O'Neil, 2008). This means that entrepreneurial investment for these clinics will require both patience and available capital to sustain these clinics until they reach profitability (Scott, 2006; Costello, 2008).

Profitability

Under the "host" model, retailers and the companies that own and operate retail clinics within the retail establishments must achieve profits. This is a unique requirement that characterizes their relationship. If either party does not see profitability, it can exit the relationship. Retailers typically operate with slim margins, which cause them to maximize the productivity of their asset. For example, retailers often use space such as waiting areas near pharmacies or vending machine areas that generate less income per square foot than the clinics are expected to provide (Scott, 2006).

With the trend toward retail pharmacy-owned clinic companies, the clinic's ability to make a profit may be enhanced by the parent company that seeks new business for the clinics. For example, Take Care Health Systems, which is owned by Walgreens, is exploring relationships with employers such as Toyota Corporation. The revised retail clinic model in which the clinic is owned by the retailer will offer a new source of revenue. The pharmacy business or hospital benefits from downstream business that flows from the clinic.

Do They Satisfy Consumer Needs for Quality Care?

Data from an early 2007 Harris Interactive Poll reported that consumers are satisfied overall with retail clinics, but especially satisfied with quality of care. Satisfaction was measured in terms of convenience (83 percent satisfied), cost (80 percent satisfied), qualifications of staff (80 percent satisfied), and quality of care (93 percent satisfied) (CVS Caremark, 2008; Harris Interactive, 2008).

Clinic operators have demonstrated achievement of a number of quality indicators. For example, MinuteClinics became the first clinic operator to be certified by the Joint Commission, which accredits health care organizations (CVS Caremark, 2008). The Minnesota Community Measurement Health Care Quality Report (2006) reported that MinuteClinics scored high marks on quality measures, in some cases scoring higher than the Mayo Clinic in certain quality dimensions. For example, in the treatment of sore throats, each clinic was evaluated on the basis of whether they administered a strep test and prescribed antibiotics only if there was a positive test result. MinuteClinics scored 100 percent, while the Mayo Clinic scored only 74 percent (Daily Policy Digest, 2006). In 2007, James Woodburn, M.D. and chief medical officer for MinuteClinics, offered that during the past five years, its clinics had treated nearly 800,000 patients without a single malpractice complaint (Basler, 2007, p. 13).

The Convenient Care Association, the retail clinic industry's trade group, also offers guidelines and standards in a variety of areas, including infection control, data collection, use of technology, and maintaining relationships with other providers, including hospitals and physicians (Deloitte, 2008). There may be structural advantages that enable retail clinics to maintain close relationships with these providers because of their use of electronic medical records (Litch, 2008).

Quality of care has been the focal point of most concern and skepticism, especially by the physicians. However, consider that many people delay or postpone seeking care because it is not affordable or because they cannot get an appointment. Instead, they often self-diagnose and self-treat, using over-the-counter medications. Thus it would seem that a visit to a retail health care clinic would be preferable to delaying treatment.

The cofounder of Take Care Health, Hal Rosenbluth offers additional support for the use of non-physician clinicians. Nurse practitioners are sanctioned to practice full primary care in rural areas where there are shortages of physicians. They are also deemed good enough to treat American soldiers in war zones such as Iraq, often performing emergency services such as tracheotomies. If nurse practitioners are competent to perform on their own in these challenging environments, they should be similarly capable of providing basic care services without physician oversight (Merchant Medicine, 2009a).

Because of advances in diagnostic and therapeutic technologies, nurse practitioners and others can now competently and reliably diagnose and treat illnesses and oversee disease management. Additionally, because the cost of physician services is high relative to nurse practitioners, the less expensive nurse practitioner can afford to spend additional time with the patient. Even though there are a lot of factors that influence quality, the ability of a nurse practitioner to spend an extra ten minutes with each patient must count for something (Christensen, Bohmer, & Kenagy, 2000; Sage, 2007).

Most of the retail clinics use standardized protocols and electronic medical records. In the case of MinuteClinics, they reportedly invested $15 million in software that incorporates clinical guidelines established by medical journals and professional academies. Of course, the clinics offer physician backup through email or the telephone (Andrews, 2004; Spencer, 2005).

Finally, physician criticism of these retail health care clinics is at odds with what is occurring elsewhere in medicine. Patients increasingly are beginning to receive some of their medical services outside the traditional physician office setting through email or telephone consultations (Herrick, 2006; Stengle, 2005). Physician entrepreneurs have also developed prototype models of retail clinics featuring nurse practitioners. In some cases, physicians are managing these enterprises for retailers such as Walmart (Jack-ovics, 2005; Rowland, 2005).

HOW DO RETAIL CLINICS "FIT" WITH HEALTH CARE REFORM EFFORTS?

The PricewaterhouseCoopers Health Research Institute's predic-tions for the top eight issues that will affect the health care industry in the future include the pressure that the growth of retail clinics will put on states, payers, and policy makers to improve the deliv-ery of primary care (Kaisernetwork, 2008a). For example, retail clinics offer a product that meets the needs of the uninsured and the underinsured—affordable basic health services. Given that the uninsured is a major concern of health reform, legislators and pol-icy makers would do well to consider the potential of retail clinics to assist in helping meet the needs of the uninsured.

Researchers from the Rand Study suggested that retail clinics perform almost as a safety net for the uninsured (Mehrotra et al., 2008). And a study of family use of retail clinics reported that unin-sured families accounted for 27 percent of retail clinic visits (Tu & Cohen, 2008). Where will the uninsured go for care if there are no retail clinics?

Walmart publicly explains how its retail clinics meet the needs of the uninsured and underscores the fact that if it were not for retail clinics, many of the uninsured would go untreated. The following statement appears on the Walmart Web site:

> Help for the uninsured
> Our retail clinics are an especially valuable resource for individuals without health insurance. Nearly half of all clinic patients report that they are uninsured. Many visitors have said that if it were not for our clinics, they wouldn't have gotten care—or they would've had to go to an emergency room. By visiting one of our clinics, patients receive the care they need and at the same time reduce overcrowding in emergency rooms and eliminate the costs of unnecessary hospital visits. (Walmart Stores, 2009)

Walgreens announced plans to offer free retail clinic visits to the unemployed and uninsured during 2009. The retailer will use its Take Care Health clinics to provide tests and routine treatments for minor ailments. Patients will still pay for prescriptions. Quest Diagnostics, a medical lab operator is also participating by offering free tests for strep throat and urinary tract infections. Walgreens is not certain how much the free services will cost the company. Take Care Health Systems estimates it has seen about 1.2 million patients since 2005 when it was launched. Approximately 30 percent of those patients were uninsured (Yahoo News, 2009).

The Downside

Retail clinics could ultimately help to reduce health care costs as well as overcrowded emergency rooms and physician offices, but there is a downside. They are also breaking apart or unbundling basic medical care with the potential to *cherry-pick* the most profitable services. This would leave the least-profitable services to existing providers of basic medical care, reduce their market share and profitability, and threaten their long-term survival.

If retail clinics are profitable, they will continue to proliferate and provide care for many who currently have no source of care or insurance. They will also likely move on to offer additional types of care beyond basic primary services. Chronic care and well care seem to be two markets that would be a fit with the retail concept. Because of the diverse nature of health services, retailers will avoid critically ill patients with complex diseases that require specialized care. But chronic and basic care needs represent potential growth markets for them.

But what happens if they are not profitable, if the business model fails, or if the clinics experience adverse events and malpractice lawsuits? Without these clinics, where will patients go? In the 1970s and 1980s, for-profit hospital companies abandoned communities when they could not make a profit. They simply closed or sold off the hospital as an asset. They left town and moved on to the next market. The decision was strictly a business one. Even when the for-profit companies stayed in town, they often discontinued unprofitable service lines at hospitals, including closing emergency departments. During the recession, we have seen nonprofit hospitals make similar business decisions to reduce or eliminate services, especially care for the poor and uninsured.

Some might say that retail clinics can potentially disappear if they are not profitable. This possibility makes an argument for a government health plan and a guaranteed safety net. But a government health care program will be ineffective if we continue to experience shortages of health professionals, especially primary care physicians. The Commmonwealth Fund survey (2006), "Public Views on U.S. Health System Organization: A Call for New

Directions," reported that 73 percent of people have had difficulty getting access to their doctor when they needed to. Sixty percent said it was difficult to get care on weekends or in the evenings from their regular doctor, so they end up in the emergency room (Schoen et al., 2006).

A survey of primary care physicians in 2006 found that only 40 percent had any kind of after-hour arrangements. The majority of physicians are in small practices with only a few doctors. If doctors want to extend their evening and weekend hours, they likely will be working all of the time (Andrews, 2008).

WHAT DOES THE FUTURE PREDICT FOR RETAIL CLINICS?

The impact of the retail clinic is potentially very substantial. It includes lower costs for services, increased access to primary care especially for the uninsured and underinsured, increased convenience for the customer, and perhaps a solution for the shortage of primary care physicians. Even though these clinics may appeal to consumers, they directly challenge existing models of physician directed care that have prevailed in the United States for over a century (Winkenwerder, 2008).

Is health care going retail? There is a spectrum of retail health care. At one end are the retail clinics, which represent low cost care. At the opposite end, there is concierge care. Concierge care is a high end concept that offers highly personalized services and guaranteed appointments for patients who are willing to pay an extra fee for these services. Some entrepreneurs such as former AOL founder Steve Case have invested in both types of care, including a network of retail clinics, RediClinics, and a health concierge service (Knott, Ahlquist, & Edmunds, 2007).

Will Retail Clinics Continue to Grow?

There is little agreement on the future of retail clinics among industry analysts and researchers. Both opponents and proponents of retail clinics can point to evidence supporting their case (Costello, 2008, p. 1300). The Rand Corporation study (Mehrotra et al., 2008) predicted growth of these clinics, reaching 6,000 by 2011. Their source was a California HealthCare Foundation Study prepared by an industry expert, Mary Kate Scott (Scott, 2006). The Convenience Care Association projected that the number of clinics would also grow to 6,000 by 2012 (Fenn, 2008).

Yet a 2008 study funded by the Robert Wood Johnson Foundation has challenged the Rand study's growth expectations (Tu & Cohen, 2008). In addition, Merchant Medicine, a source of industry news concerning retail clinics, also believes that 6,000 clinics by 2012 is probably too high a projection. However, they do expect that there will continue to be growth among retail clinics (Merchant Medicine, 2009a). Tom Charland, president and CEO of Merchant Medicine predicted that there could be as many as 3,000 retail clinics nationwide by 2013, and that these clinics will each see approximately 8,000 patient visits per clinic per year. Charland has been a key player in retail clinics, having previously served as senior vice president of strategy and business development at MinuteClinics (Litch, 2008, p. 31).

Despite this conflicting evidence about the future of retail clinics, it is conceivable that a slowdown in growth simply represents the natural evolution of a new business model (Costello, 2008). However, there is no evidence that Walmart is slowing down. Although 23 of its stores saw clinics close in 2008, 80 clinics remained open (Goldstein, 2008). Furthermore, Walmart executives maintain that they still plan to lease space to several hundred clinics during the next two years and to offer space to as many as 2,000 clinics by 2014. Walmart is particularly interested in adding more hospital-linked retail clinics (Freudenheim, 2009).

Retail clinics may be predictive of the future design of the delivery of primary care in the United States: niche service markets. These clinics reflect an operating system in which all elements, from location, to information systems, to staffing, to clinical and business processes, as well as to range of services, are intentionally aligned to meet the needs of a specific group of consumers, the less sick. By focusing on this small segment of the population, the less sick, retail clinics may free up primary care visits for those with more complex medical problems, thereby reducing crowded doctors' offices and appointment calendars as well as emergency departments (Bohmer, 2007, p. 767–768).

Survivability

However, the larger question remains regarding the future of retail clinics: Will they be profitable? If the clinics are not profitable, retailers will look for other means of entering health care markets. Because retail clinics are capital intensive, they take time to return a profit. Many private investors that initially backed retail clinic operators thought that they could make a quick return off of their investment. They were not prepared for a long-term commitment. Smart Care, one of the privately backed retail clinic operators that closed, saw investors exit before clinics were launched (Merchant Medicine, 2009c). But retailers and large investors and entrepreneurs such as Richard Scott (Solantic) and Steven Case (Redi-Clinics) appear to still be in the game and willing to continue to revise their business models to achieve success.

Retail clinics have a short history in health care. Yet because of the "fast" nature of the retail industry, they have undergone an accelerated evolution of growth and development in search of profitability. The early "host" model in which retailers leased store space to privately backed clinic operators, still exists, but there have been some revisions to the model. Larger pharmacy retailers have transitioned to owners of clinic companies through acquisition and have shifted from opening new clinics to also developing new markets, products, and services such as pharmacy benefits management programs with self-insured employers (Merchant Medicine, 2009d). Furthermore, the growth of hospital-linked retail clinics bears watching as hospitals have discovered that these clinics perform as feeder systems for them (Freudenheim, 2009).

As retailers continue to search for new markets, they likely will include employers who are eager to reduce costs. For example, Walgreens is marketing a combination of its services, from clinics to pharmacies, to help businesses save on employee health care costs. Two programs, Complete Care and Well-Being, are aimed at cutting employers' health care and prescription costs. These programs offer employees services at in-store clinics and also at business sites (Wohl & Zimmerman, 2009). Walmart is also testing an employer model to reduce prescription drug prices for employers much the way Walmart cut prescription prices for consumers in 2006 (Jones, 2009).

As long as the health care needs and wants of Americans exceed their ability and willingness to pay, there is an opening for Walmart and other low-cost providers to fill the gap. Such a change would significantly impact health care labor markets, survivability of existing competitors, quality of care, quality of service, and clinical outcomes. Retailers are expected to capture the most profitable market segments, leaving the least-profitable primary care services to existing competitors, reduce their market share and profitability, and threaten their long-term survival.

Putting Consumers First

The early success of retail health care clinics shows that patients are amenable to receive treatment outside of traditional settings because it is quick, affordable, and convenient. More importantly, retail clinics have not been shown to disrupt the patient-physician relationship. Most who visit retail clinics have no regular source of care (Mehrotra et al., 2008).

In *Money Driven Medicine* (2006), author Maggie Mahar suggests that the purchase of health care is different from other purchases because the transaction is based on trust and the belief that the physician will put the patients' interests first. This is contrary to what occurs among corporate retailers who may put their shareholders' interests ahead of their customers.

> Corporate retailers such as Wal-Mart and McDonald's are expected to be honest, but they are not expected to be selfless; they are not expected to put their customers' interests ahead of their shareholders'. But physicians are not retailers, and health care is not a retail industry or even a service industry in the ordinary sense of the term. (Mahar, 2006, pp. 343–344)

Given the trend toward retail clinics, especially, hospital-linked retail clinics, the nature of the health care industry may be changing.

REFERENCES

Alsever, J. (2004, April 25). In-store back-pain clinics ride on shoulders of Wal-Mart. *The Denver Post*, pp. 1k–8k.

Andrews, M. (2004, July 18). *Next to the express checkout, express medical care*. Retrieved November 4, 2005, from The New York Times Official Site: www.nytimes.com.

Andrews, M. (2005, February 1). *Gone in 60 seconds: An innovative chain called MinuteClinic is trying to reinvent the way you get treated for routine ailments*. Retrieved November 4, 2005, from CNN Money.com Official Site, Fortune Small Business: http://money.cnn.com/magazines/fsb/fsb_archive/2005/02/01/8250649/index.htm.

Andrews, M. (2008, August 7). *Where to turn for immediate medical care*. Retrieved November 11, 2008, from U.S. News: http://health.usnews.com/blogs/on-health-and-money/2008/08/07/where-to-turn-for-immediate-medical-care.html.

Associated Press. (2007, August 11). *Health clinics expand in retail settings*. Retrieved August 13, 2007, from BostonHerald.com: http://www

.bostonherald.com/business/healthcare/view.bg?articleid=10166
91&srvc=next.

Associated Press. (2008). *Wal-Mart to open in-store medical clinics.* Retrieved
February 7, 2008, from MSNBC.com: http://www.msnbc.msn.com/
id/23048157/.

Basler, B. (2007, April 12). Care in the express lane. *AARP Bulletin, 48*(4),
12–14.

Bazzoli, F. (2008). *Cigna agreement expands retail clinic coverage
option.* Retrieved March 13, 2008, from Healthcarefinance News:
http://www.healthcarefinancenews.com/news/cigna-agreement-
expands-retail-clinic-coverage-option.

Bergdahl, M. (2004). *What I learned from Sam Walton: How to compete and
thrive in a Wal-Mart.* Hoboken, NJ: John Wiley & Sons, Inc.

Bohmer, R. (2007). The rise of in-store clinics—Threats or opportunity?
The New England Journal of Medicine, 356(8), 765–768.

Bowling, K. (2007). *Solantic founder Richard L. Scott given prestigous entre-
prenurial award from the George Washington University.* Retrieved
May 12, 2009, from Solantic: http://www.solantic.com/press/scott
%20gw%20release%20nov%202007.pdf.

Bowman, D. (2008). *Common retail clinic locations.* Retrieved June 12,
2008, from FierceHealthcare: http://www.fiercehealthcare.com/
slideshows/common-retail-clinic-locations?img=1.

Christensen, C. M., Bohmer, R., & Kenagy, J. (2000, September 1). Will disruptive innovations cure health care? *Harvard Business Review,*
Reprint R00501, 1–9.

Consumer Reports. (2009, April). When you need care fast. *Consumer
Reports on Health,* 6.

Costello, D. (2008). Report from the field—A checkup for retail medicine.
Health Affairs, 27(5), 1299–1303.

CVS Caremark. (2008). *MinuteClinic receives JCAHO accreditation.*
Retrieved March 1, 2009, from CVS Caremark: http://investor
.cvs.com/phoenix.zhtml?c=99533&p=irol-newsarticle&id=907392.

Daily, L. (2006, March/April). Say "Ah" in aisle 3—At a retailer near you:
on-the-spot medical care. *AARP Magazine,* 22.

Daily Policy Digest. (2006, November). *MinuteClinic scores high marks on
quality measures.* Retrieved December 6, 2006, from National Center
for Policy Analysis, Daily Policy Digest—Patient Power Pulse:
http://www.ncpa.org/sub/dpd/index.php?article_id=13900.

Deloitte. (2008). *Retail medical clinics: Disrupting models of primary care.*
Retrieved November 13, 2008, from Deloitte: http://www.deloitte
.com/dtt/article/0,1002,sid%253d127087%2526cid%253d217872,00
.html.

Denning, A. (2006). *America's family physicians urge retail health clinics to
put patients' health first.* Retrieved December 11, 2006, from The
American Academy of Family Physicians: http://www.aafp.org/
online/en/home/media/releases/2006/20060622retailhlth.html.

Dentzer, S. (2008). Innovations: "Medical home" or medical motel 6? *Health Affairs, 27*(5), 1216–1217.

Fenn, S. (2008). Integrating CCCs into the Hospital System. *Frontiers of Health Services Management, 24*(3), 33–36.

FierceHealthcare. (June 6, 2007a). *New retail clinic services air travelers.* Retrieved June 12, 2008, from FierceHealthcare Official Site: http://www.fiercehealthcare.com/node/5658/print.

FierceHealthcare. (January 1, 2007b). *Retail clinics keep advancing.* Retrieved June 12, 2008, from FierceHealthcare Official Site: http://www.fiercehealthcare.com/node/4534/print.

FierceHealthcare. (April 8, 2008a). *Airport clinics, pharmacies become more common.* Retrieved June 12, 2008, from FierceHealthcare Official Site: http://www.fiercehealthcare.com/node/23494/print.

FierceHealthcare. (June 4, 2008b). *FTC comes down on IL bill restricting retail clinics.* Retrieved June 4, 2008, from FierceHealthcare Official Site: http://www.fiercehealthcare.com/story/ftc-comes-down-on-il-bill-restricting-retail-clinics/2008-06-04.

FierceHealthcare. (January 10, 2008c). *MA sets retail clinic rules.* Retrieved June 12, 2008, from FierceHealthcare Official Site: http://www.fiercehealthcare.com/node/14815/print.

FierceHealthcare. (January 30, 2008d). *Start-up closes 23 Wal-Mart retail clinics.* Retrieved June 3, 2008, from FierceHealthcare Official Site: http://www.fiercehealthcare.com/node/16513/print.

FierceHealthcare. (January 16, 2008e). *Study: Retail clinics at about 1,000 in U.S.* Retrieved January 16, 2008, from FierceHealthcare Official Site: http://www.fiercehealthcare.com/node/15265/print.

FierceHealthcare. (February 8, 2008f). *Wal-Mart Plans its own in-store clinics.* Retrieved June 12, 2008, from FierceHealthcare Official Site: http://www.fiercehealthcare.com/node/17567/print.

Fineman, J. (2006). *Wal-Mart, CVS alarm doctors as retailers push clinics (Update 2).* Retrieved November 10, 2008, from Bloomberg.com: http://bloomberg.com/apps/news?pid=20601109&sid=atboick4bsd4&refer=news.

Freudenheim, M. (2006, May 14). *Attention shoppers: Low prices on shots in clinic.* Retrieved November 10, 2008, from *The New York Times*: http://www.nytimes.com/2006/05/14/business/14clinic.html?sq=attention%20shoppers:%20low%20prices%20on%20shots%20in%20clinic&st=cse&scp=1&pagewanted=print.

Freudenheim, M. (2009, May 12). *Hospitals begin to move into supermarkets.* Retrieved May 12, 2009, from *The New York Times*: http://www.nytimes.com/2009/05/12/business/12clinic.html.

Gammon, K. S. (2007). *Docs split on big-box clinics—Debate rages over convenience, cost and quality concerns.* Retrieved June 27, 2007, from ABC News: http://abcnews.go.com/print?id=3319003.

Gentry, C. (2007). *Coalition pushes transparency in medical costs.* Retrieved June 22, 2007, from TBO.com, Tampa Bay Online: http://www2

.tbo.com/content/2007/jun/19/bz-coalition-pushes-transparency-in-medical-costs/.

Goldstein, J. (2008). *Wal-Mart clinics close in 23 stores*. Retrieved January 30, 2008, from *The Wall Street Journal*: http://blogs.wsj.com/health/2008/01/29/wal-mart-clinics-close-in-23-stores/?mod=homeblog mod_healthb.

Good Housekeeping. (2008, September). Visit your drugstore's clinic. *Good Housekeeping*, 52.

Harris Interactive. (2008). *Harris Interactive restructures US operations to improve profits and promote growth*. Retrieved December 29, 2008, from Harris Interactive: http://www.harrisinteractive.com/news/allnewsbydate.asp?newsid1201.

Herrick, D. (2006, January 1). *Demand growing for corporate practice of medicine*. Retrieved December 31, 2005, from The Heartland Institute: http://www.heartland.org/publications/health%20care/article/18269/demand_growing_for_corporate_practice_of_medicine.html.

Herzlinger, R. E. (2006, August 29). Why innovation in health care is so hard. *Harvard Buisness Review, 84*(5), 58–66.

Honaman, C. J. (2006, November/December). Going retail—New leadership skills to keep up with healthcare's market shift. *Healthcare Executive*, 49–50.

Immediate Care Business. (2009). *Cleveland Clinic teams with Minute-Clinic*. Retrieved February 21, 2009, from Immediate Care Business Official Site: http://www.immediatecarebusiness.com/hotnews/cleveland-clinic–minuteclinic-team-up.html#.

Jackovics, T. (2005). *It's OK now if you shop till you drop*. Retrieved January 2, 2006, from *Tampa Tribune*: http://www.tbo.com.

Japsen, B. (June 25, 2007a). *AMA takes on retail clinics—Doctors groups say patients in danger*. Retrieved June 27, 2007, from *Chicago Tribune*: http://archives.chicagotribune.com/2007/jun/25/business/chi-clinics_bizjun25.

Japsen, B. (June 30, 2007b). *American Medical Association to Fight Retail Health Clinics*. Retrieved July 2, 2007, from *Post-Bulletin*: http://postbulletin.com/newsmanager/templates/localnews_story.asp?a=299120&z=2.

Japsen, B. (2008, July 24). *In-store clinic growth slowing*. Retrieved July 24, 2008, from Chicagotribune.com: http://www.chicagotribune.com/business/chi-thu-notebook-retail-clinic-jul24,0,7722240,print.story.

Jones, S. M. (2009, March 28). *Drug prices: Wal-Mart/Caterpillar plan may drive down employer health-care costs*. Retrieved May 9, 2009, from Chicagotribune.com: http://archives.chicagotribune.com/2009/mar/28/business/chi-sat-wal-mart-pharmacy-mar28.

Kaisernetwork. (June 26, 2007a). *AMA calls on state, federal officials to investigate whether retail health clinics create conflicts of interest*. Retrieved

June 27, 2007, from Kaisernetwork: http://www.kaisernetwork .org/daily_reports/print_report.cfm?dr_id=45835&dr_cat=3.

Kaisernetwork. (June 27, 2007b). *AMA should not seek to "stifle" retail health clinics, editorial states.* Retrieved June 27, 2007, from Kaiser Daily Health Policy Report—Kaisernetwork.org: http://www.kaiser network.org/daily_reports/print_report.cfm?DR_ID=45880&dr _cat=3.

Kaisernetwork. (November 14, 2007c). *Coverage & access | Some medical centers open facilities to compete with retail medical clinics.* Retrieved May 20, 2008, from Kaisernetwork: http://www.kaisernetwork .org/daily_reports/rep_index.cfm?hint=3&dr_id=48863.

Kaisernetwork. (May 21, 2007d). *Medical community questions nationwide expansion of retail clinics.* Retrieved May 23, 2007, from Kaiser Daily Health Policy Report—Kaisernetwork.org: http://www.kaisernet work.org/daily_reports/print_report.cfm?DR_ID=45040&dr _cat=3.

Kaisernetwork. (March 13, 2007e). *Number of retail clinics continues to increase, analysts say.* Retrieved June 12, 2008, from Kaiser Daily Health Policy Report—Kaisernetwork.org: http://www .kaisernetwork.org/daily_reports/print_report.cfm?DR_ID=43551 &dr_cat=3.

Kaisernetwork. (May 14, 2007f). *Retail clinics offer U.S. residents more accessible, affordable health care, opinion piece states.* Retrieved May 23, 2007, from Kaiser Daily Health Policy Report—Kaisernetwork.org: http://www.kaisernetwork.org/daily_reports/print_report.cfm? DR_ID=44899&dr_cat=3.

Kaisernetwork. (February 6, 2007g). *Retail health clinic trade group expects number of clinics to double by end of year.* Retrieved June 12, 2008, from Kaiser Daily Health Policy Report, Kaisernetwork.org: http:// www.kaisernetwork.org/daily_reports/print_report.cfm?dr_id= 42762&dr_cat=3.

Kaisernetwork. (August 9, 2007h). *Several states consider regulating in-store health clinics amid safety concerns, Wall Street Journal reports.* Retrieved June 12, 2008, from Kaiser Daily Health Policy Report— Kaisernetwork.org: http://www.kaisernetwork.org/daily_reports/ rep_index.cfm?hint=3&dr_id=46781.

Kaisernetwork. (January 16, 2008a). *Columnist examines predictions for health care industry in 2008.* Retrieved June 12, 2008, from Kaiser Daily Health Policy Report: http://www.kaisernetwork.org/daily _reports/print_report.cfm?dr_id=49863&dr_cat=3.

Kaisernetwork. (May 7, 2008b). *Some operators closing retail clinics, scaling back expansion plans.* Retrieved June 12, 2008, from Kaiser Daily Health Policy Report, Kaisernetwork.org: http://www.kaisernet work.org/daily_reports/print_report.cfm?dr_id=52002&dr_cat=3.

Keckley, P., Underwood, H. R., & Gandhi, M. (2008). *Retail clinics: Facts, trends and implications, Deloitte Center for Health Solutions.*

Retrieved April 5, 2009, from Deloitte Official Site: http://www2.deloitte.com/assets/Dcom-UnitedStates/local%20Assets/Documents/us_chs_RetailClinics_230708.pdf.

Kershaw, S. (2007). *Drugstore clinics spread, and scrutiny grows.* Retrieved August 23, 2007, from *The New York Times*: http://www.nytimes.com/2007/08/23/nyregion/23clinic.html?scp=1&sq=the%20concept%20has%20been%20called%20urgent%20care%20%22lite%22&st=cse.

Knott, D., Ahlquist, G., & Edmunds, R. (2007). *Health care's retail solution.* Retrieved May 14, 2007, from Strategy+Business: http://strategy-business.com/press/article/07107?pg=all&tid+230.

Kowalczyk, L. (2009). *Sick flocking to in-store clinics—Convenience draws patients to CVS, but doctors' reaction mixed.* Retrieved March 14, 2009, from *The Boston Globe*: http://www.boston.com/news/health/articles/2009/03/12/sick_flocking_to_in_store_clinics/.

Ladue, C. (2008). *Number of retail health clinics nearing 1,000 nationwide.* Retrieved January 16, 2008, from Healthcare Finance News: http://healthcarefinancenews.com/story.cms?id=7520.

Langston, E. (2007). *The AMA's work for doctors and patients.* Retrieved August 2, 2007, from Washingtonpost.com: http://www.washingtonpost.com/wp-dyn/content/article/2007/07/27/AR2007072702049.html.

Laws, M., & Scott, K. (2008, September/October). The emergence of retail-based clinics in the United States: Early observations. *Health Affairs, 27*(5), 1293–1298.

Lebhar-Friedman. (2006). *Retail clinician—Drug store news announces the launch of a new professional publication "Retail Clinician."* Retrieved December 6, 2006, from Marketwire: http://www.marketwire.com/press-release/lebhar-friedman-685144.html.

Lee, P. V., & Lansky, D. (2008). Perspective—Making space for disruption: Putting patients at the center of health care. *Health Affairs, 27*(5), 1345–1348.

Levy, M. (2006). *Rite Aid's in-store health clinics close in Ore.* Retrieved December 6, 2006, from Mercury News: http://www.mercurynews.com/mld/mercurynews/news/breaking_news/15644510.htm?template=contentm.

Litch, B. (2008, September/October). Retail clinics: Making the decision to join the game. *Healthcare Executive, 23*(5), 27–33.

Lohr, S. (2009, March 11). Wal-Mart plans to market digital health records system. *The New York Times*, p. B1.

Mahar, M. (2006). *Money driven medicine.* New York: Harper Collins Publishers.

Mehrotra, A., Wang, M. C., Lave, J. R., Adams, J. L., & McGlynn, E. A. (2008, September/October). Retail clinics, primary care physicians, and emergency departments: A comparison of patients' visits. *Health Affairs, 27*(5), 1272–1282.

Merchant Medicine. (2008). *Feature: Retail clinics and primary care, will the scope of care always be simple episodic illnesses?*. Retrieved November 11, 2008, from Merchant Medicine: http://www.merchantmedicine.com/Home.cfm.

Merchant Medicine. (April 2, 2009a). *A travel industry giant drops in on healthcare: A profile of Hal Rosenbluth*. Retrieved April 7, 2009, from Merchant Medicine: http://www.merchantmedicine.com/news.cfm?view=36.

Merchant Medicine. (April 2, 2009b). *Key factors in retail clinic growth.* Retrieved April 7, 2009, from Merchant Medicine: http://www.merchantmedicine.com/news.cfm?view=24.

Merchant Medicine. (April 2, 2009c). *Primary care meets private investor: Former retail clinic operators share lessons learned.* Retrieved April 7, 2009, from Merchant Medicine: http://www.merchantmedicine.com/news.cfm?view=29.

Merchant Medicine. (April 2, 2009d). *Retail Clinics: 2008 Year-end review and 2009 outlook: Many closures in 2008 but the market continues to expand.* Retrieved April 7, 2009, from Merchant Medicine: http://www.merchantmedicine.com/news.cfm?view=21.

Merchant Medicine. (April 2, 2009e). *Retail clinics and the changing primary care landscape.* Retrieved April 7, 2009, from Merchant Medicine: http://www.merchantmedicine.com/news.cfm?view=25.

Merchant Medicine. (March 1, 2009f). *Retail clinics by metro area: A geographic look at clinic saturation and demand.* Retrieved April 7, 2009, from Merchant Medicine: http://www.merchantmedicine.com/news.cfm?view=40. (Full PDF, Volume 2, No. 4.)

Miller, M. C. (2004, September 27). We all need a dose of the doctor: The healing relationship between patient and physician plays a vital role in medical care. *Newsweek,* 63–64.

Modern Healthcare. (2008, January 9). *Mass. panel sets rules for limited-care clinics.* Retrieved January 15, 2008, from ModernHealthcare.com: http://www.modernhealthcare.com/apps/pbcs.dll/article?aid=/20080109/reg/354323897&nocache=1&nocache=1.

Newbold, P., & O'Neil, M. J. (2008). Small changes lead to large effects. *Frontiers of Health Services Management, 24*(3), 23–27.

Pauly, M. V. (2008, September/October). Perspective—"We aren't quite as good, but we sure are cheap": Prospects for disruptive innovation in medical care and insurance markets. *Health Affairs, 27*(5), 1349–1352.

Perin, M. (2008, August 1). *Retail health clinics reopen with new model.* Retrieved February 3, 2009, from *Houston Business Journal*: http://houston.bizjournals.com/houston/stories/2008/08/04/story4.html?t=printable.

Perry, M. (2008). *Retail healthcare clinics offering most convenient solution*. Retrieved December 2, 2008, from Seeking Alpha: http://seekingalpha.com/article/79631-retail-healthcare-clinics-offering-most-convenient-solutions?source.

Porter, S. (2008). *Expect retail health clinics to expand scope of practice—Q&A with health care consultant, researcher Mary Kate Scott*. Retrieved February 3, 2009, from American Academy of Family Physicians, AAFP News Now: http://www.aafp.org/online/en/home/publications/news/news-now/professional-issues/20080723retail-q-a.html.

PRN Newswire. (2005). *PRN and the Cleveland Clinic team up to provide health tips on the Wal-Mart TV*. Retrieved July 28, 2005, from PRN.com: http://www.prn.com/about/clevelandclinicrelease.htm.

Ramachandran, N. (2006, May 1). A shot in the arm for retailers—Convenient clinics offer quick care for patients and added traffic for stores. *U.S. News & World Report*, 52–53.

Rice, B. (2005). *In-store clinics: Should you worry?* . Retrieved December 31, 2005, from Medical Economics: http://medicaleconomics.modern medicine.com/memag/article/articleDetail.jsp?id=179078.

Robinson, J. C., & Smith, M. D. (2008, September/October). Perspective—Cost-reducing innovation in health care. *Health Affairs, 27*(5), 1353–1356.

Rowland, C. (2005). *I'll have a loaf of bread, milk, and a flu shot: Discount stores*. Retrieved January 2, 2006, from *The Boston Globe*: http://www.boston.com/business/articles/2005/12/11/ill_have_a_loaf_of_bread_milk_and_a_flu_shot/.

Sage, W. M. (2007). The Wal-Martization of health care. *The Journal of Legal Medicine, 28*, 503–519.

Schoen, C., How, S. K., Weinbaum, I., Craig, J. E., & Davis, K. (2006). Public views on shaping the future of the U.S. health system. *The Commonwealth Fund, 31*, 1.

Schreiner, B. (2005). *Humana pitching Medicare plan at Wal-Mart*. Retrieved July 25, 2005, from biz.yahoo.com: http://biz.yahoo.com/ap/050713/humana_medicare.html?.v=2.

Scott, M. (2006). Health care in the express lane: The emergence of retail clinics. *Report prepared for the California Healthcare Foundation*.

Scott, M. K. (2007). *Health care in the express lane: Retail clinics go mainstream*. Retrieved May 11, 2008, from California HealthCare Foundation: http://www.chcf.org/topics/view.cfm?itemid=133464.

Senior Journal. (2007). *In-store health clinics grow as does satisfaction but not customers*. Retrieved June 27, 2007, from SeniorJournal.com: http://www.seniorjournal.com/news/features/2007/7-04-18-in-store.htm.

Smith, S. (January 9, 2008a). *In-store clinics approved*. Retrieved February 12, 2008, from The Boston Globe Official Site: http://www.boston .com/news/health/blog/2008/01/instore_clinics.html.

Smith, S. (January 11, 2008b). *Menino decries clinics in retailers—Urges health council to bar infirmaries from opening in city.* Retrieved February 12, 2008, from *The Boston Globe*: http://www.boston.com/news/ local/articles/2008/01/11/menino_decries_clinics_in_retailers/.

Smith, S. (June 12, 2008c). *Walgreens plans clinics to rival CVS's*. Retrieved June 12, 2008, from *The Boston Globe*: http://www.boston.com/ business/healthcare/articles/2008/06/12/walgreens_plans_clinics _to_rival_cvss/.

Spencer, J. (2005). Getting your healthcare at Wal-Mart. *Wall Street Journal, 266*(70), D1–D5.

Starr, P. (1982). *The social transformation of American medicine*. New York: Basic Books.

Stengle, J. (2005, December 3). Telephone doctor service giving critics headaches: Patients get advice without exams. *The Tampa Tribune, Nation/World*, p. 10.

Tu, H. T., & Cohen, G. R. (2008). Checking up on retail-based health clinics: Is the boom ending? *The Commonwealth Fund, 48*, 1–12.

Turner, G. (2007, May 14). Customer health care. *The Wall Street Journal*, p. A17.

Walmart Stores. (2007). *Dr. John Agwunobi to join Wal-Mart as Senior Vice President and President for the Professional Services Division*. Retrieved December 11, 2008, from Walmartstores.com: http://walmart stores.com/FactsNews/NewsRoom/6654.aspx.

Wal-mart Stores. (2009). *Clinics*. Retrieved February 3, 2009, from Walmartstores.com: http://Wal-Martstores.com/healthwellness/ 7613.aspx?gclid=copp77cdwzgcfrwwawodcj.

The Wall Street Journal. (2007). *Drugstore clinics and the convenience kerfuffle*. Retrieved August 20, 2007, from *The Wall Street Journal* Official Site: http://online.wsj.com/article/SB118740056581701633.html.

Wohl, J., & Zimmerman, D. (2009, January 14). *Walgreen offers health program for businesses*. Retrieved January 14, 2009, from Reuters.com: http://www.reuters.com/article/idustre50d4vj20090114.

Woznicki, K. (2004). *Growing number of big stores featuring quick-fix medical clinics*. Retrieved January 2, 2006, from MedPage: http://www .medpagetoday.com/PublicHealthPolicy/PracticeManagement/ 1933.

Wild, R. (2006, July/August). Your take-charge guide to affordable health care. *AARP The Magazine*, 51–55, 75.

Winkenwerder, W. (2008). *Retail medical clinics: Here to stay?* Retrieved November 13, 2008, from Deloitte: http://www.deloitte.com/dtt/ article/0,1002,sid%253d127087%2526cid%253d192739,00.html.

Yahoo News. (2009, March 31). *Walgreens giving free care to jobless and uninsured*. Retrieved April 22, 2009, from Yahoo News: http://news.yahoo.com.

Yu, R. (2008). *Health care businesses take off at airports*. Retrieved April 8, 2008, from *USA Today*: http://www.usatoday.com/travel/flights/2008-04-07-airport-clinics-pharmacies_n.htm.

Chapter 6

Retail Clinic Demographics and Performance

In this chapter we will review the demographic characteristics of those consumers who utilize retail health clinics. We will also assess data relevant to the performance of these clinics. Such data include case study data as well as consumer and expert perceptions of various service attributes. Among the performance measures we will assess regarding retail health clinics are access, relative costs, quality of care, patient satisfaction, financial viability, and transparency/accountability.

DEMOGRAPHIC CHARACTERISTICS OF RETAIL CLINIC USERS

Previous research has shown that retail clinic users are younger than nonusers. However, users are not significantly different in terms of their health status from nonusers. Previous research has also found that the rates of users and nonusers of retail clinics were similar in terms of their sickness and drug usage (Forrester Research, 2007).

Table 6.1 provides a summary of retail clinic user demographics for MinuteClinic, which is a major clinic provider of health services in retail settings. It is clear from the table that retail clinics serve a high percentage of non-whites, low income families, young people, the uninsured, and those without a primary care physician.

The 2008 survey of health care consumers by Deloitte found that consumers with the following characteristics were interested and more likely to potentially use retail clinics:

TABLE 6.1   Demographic Characteristics of Retail Clinic Users

• Equal split between male and female

• 40 percent are non-white (vs. 18 percent for nonusers)

• 28 percent have less than $40,000 household income (vs. 16 percent for nonusers)

• 30 percent are between the ages of 19 and 30 (vs. 17 percent for nonusers)

• 28 percent do not have a primary physician (vs. 15 percent for nonusers)

• 12 percent are uninsured (vs. 6 percent for nonusers)

Source: Market Strategies: "MinuteClinic—The Evolving Face of Consumerism in Healthcare," October 23, 2007.

• Baby boomers were very interested, with nearly 38 percent saying they would use a retail clinic.
• Generation-Y members were the most likely to use a retail clinic.
• Seniors were least likely to use a retail clinic.
• Those in better than average health, those distrustful of hospitals and doctors, those suspicious of the medications that hospitals and doctors prescribe, and the uninsured were more likely to use a retail clinic than those with the opposite characteristics. (Deloitte Center for Health Solutions, 2008c)

In 2007 the Center for Studying Health System Change performed a "Health Tracking Household Survey" of a nationally representative sample in 9,400 families. The demographic characteristics of those families most likely to use retail clinics were as follows:

• Families not receiving any care in the previous year.
• Young families with parents between the ages of 18 and 34.
• Uninsured families.
• Hispanic and African American consumers.
• Families with no primary care physician.
• Childless families. (Tu & Cohen, 2008)

Another recent study (Mehrotra et al., 2008) found that retail clinics serve a patient population that is underserved by primary care physicians. More specifically, these authors found that females, youth, the uninsured, and patients who do not have a regular primary care doctor tended to visit retail clinics more than males, senior citizens, those with insurance, and those having a primary care physician. The latter demographic groups were more likely to utilize primary care physicians or emergency departments.

Increasingly, those who are under- and uninsured are paying for services up-front before they are rendered (Henry J. Kaiser Family Foundation, 2006). Retail clinics constitute most of these up-front expenditures. With affordable up-front, menu-style pricing, retail clinics can mean the difference between a person receiving and not receiving necessary health care services. Consumers receiving care in Walmart clinics (55 percent) do not have health insurance. These uninsured consumers as well as others without a primary care physician are provided with an entry into the health care system through Walmart clinics (Walmart Stores, 2006).

In sum, it appears that retail clinic users are those consumers who are less likely to be well served by primary care physicians, hospitals, and other traditional providers. These obviously include the uninsured and underinsured, but they also include young people, minorities, lower income groups, families with no primary care physician, childless families, and those not previously receiving care in the past year. Obviously, retail medical clinics are meeting a consumer need.

PERFORMANCE OF RETAIL HEALTH CLINICS

Access

For most time-strapped consumers, convenience is a major service attribute that is highly valued. However, our health care system is not known for providing high levels of convenience. The system's inconvenience is reflected in the long waiting times consumers experience in most of their health care encounters. Not only are consumers forced to wait for an appointment, they must also wait for physicians to open their offices, and they further wait upon their arrival to actually see the physician. The "bottom line" is that long wait times at every stage in the care process frustrates consumers because it wastes their time.

According to the Agency for Healthcare Research and Quality (2006), patients receive an appointment at a convenient time only about 52 percent of the time. In addition, they are able to see the doctor within 15 minutes of arrival only 23 percent of the time. Emergency room patients who did not have an emergency condition often wait more than an hour (Centers for Disease Control and Prevention, 2006). There is also evidence that long waiting times often result in patient dissatisfaction (BMC Health Services Research, 2007).

A major benefit of retail clinics is superior convenience because no appointments are needed, they operate during evening and weekend hours, and they offer immediate access or very short wait times. They also offer superior convenience because they are conveniently located in a variety of retail settings where consumers already shop for other goods and services. Examples include drugstores, big box retailers, and supermarkets. These locations allow consumers to multitask because they often visit them on a routine basis. Another less obvious benefit of retail clinics is that since they provide less complex care, they reduce demand for emergency room and primary care services in physician offices.

As a result of all of the above, retail clinics should gain market share of low acuity cases in the years ahead. One of the major factors driving demand for their services is the rapidly increasing number of retail clinics. Whereas Harris Interactive (2007) found that only 7 percent of U.S. consumers had experience with a retail health clinic in 2005, the Deloitte Center for Health Solutions (2008b) found that 16 percent had used such a clinic in 2008. Not only is retail clinic use increasing over time as a result of clinic availability, but the same survey (2008) found that 34 percent of consumers are willing to use them.

In one recent study (Tu & Cohen, 2008), two out of three respondents indicated the major factor in choosing a retail clinic over other sources of care was the clinic's convenient hours. The second and third highest rationales for clinic use were the convenient location and the fact that consumers did not have to make an appointment. Eighty-seven percent of clinic users identified at least one of the three above convenience factors as a major reason for patronizing retail clinics, and a third of all respondents indicated all three factors were major reasons. The likelihood of identifying hours, location, and no need for appointments as major determinants of retail clinic usage did not vary significantly across different demographic subgroups.

A former practicing primary care physician and medical group leader, Dr. William Winkenwerder, has noted the following:

> I hate to admit it, but primary care physicians have struggled to recognize a market-need in making their services conveniently available

to the busy American public. Many doctors have a difficult time accepting the notion that patients should be able to get same-day appointments or that convenient hours must include evenings and weekends. (Winkenwerder, 2009)

However, the Deloitte 2008 survey of health care consumers found 68 percent of patients would like to have access to same-day appointments at hospitals, and another 60 percent would like to be able to schedule their appointments on-line.

Retail health clinics may provide consumers with an option for gaining access to prevention and early detection health services. Health outcomes may be significantly improved through prevention and early detection. These should enhance patients' quality of life and many medical conditions as a result of appropriate screening and immunizations. In fact, the CDC has recognized that vaccination services at retail clinics offer an excellent way to expand adult vaccinations during influenza season (Centers for Disease Control, 2007). As they grow in numbers over time, retail clinics may be able to contribute to public health, epidemiology, and surveillance.

Walmart has noted the following attributes of its in-store retail clinics which enhance access for consumers:

- These clinics provide immediate access to a limited set of acute and preventive health care services to adults and children delivered by licensed, certified medical professionals who diagnose, treat, and prescribe medications in compliance with federal and state regulations.
- The clinics are open seven days a week, including nights and weekends.
- The clinics can help keep people out of overcrowded emergency rooms since 10–15 percent of clinic customers surveyed said they would have used an emergency room had the clinic in Walmart not been available. While another 5–10 percent would have gone without treatment entirely, potentially leading to more serious complications. (Walmart Stores, 2006)

Regina Herzlinger (2007), Professor at Harvard Business School, has been quite supportive of retail clinics and their ability to enhance access to health services for busy consumers:

These clinics do a lot of good. Their convenient locations and extended hours—they are usually open every day—enable ready access so that busy people need not defer important medical care such as flu shots. Their availability helps to unclog crowded emergency rooms, and their prices enable the uninsured to obtain care at reasonable costs rather than face the high prices that hospital emergency rooms too often reserve solely for the uninsured. (Herzlinger, 2007, A15)

Relative Costs

According to clinic operator Web sites (2009), the range of costs of services provided by retail clinics are typically between $50 and $75, whereas physician office visits may range from $55 to $250. Consequently, similar services provided at retail clinics may significantly reduce consumer out-of-pocket costs. An obvious example would be a physical examination which might cost from $25 to 49 in a retail setting, compared to $50–100 in a physician office. In order to gain insight into how much money health care consumers would ultimately save by going to a retail health clinic, the authors compared prices between (1) Solantic, a walk-in retail health center located in one of Walmart's stores (Orlando, Florida), and (2) a primary care physician practice also located in Orlando. The following is a list of different services provided by each of these facilities and their related costs:

Walmart's Solantic Services and Prices (3 Levels)

- Level 1: $65 includes patient visit with no diagnostic lab tests or other procedures
- Level 2: $105 includes patient visit with one procedure
- Level 3: $165 includes patient visit with two or more procedures

A few examples of what Solantic's services and prices include are as follows:

- School and/or sports physical: $25
- Employment physical: $50
- Basic checkup: $50
- Blood pressure screening: $10
- X-ray: $80
- Drug screening: $25
- MMR immunization: $75
- Hemocult: $30

Other procedures offered by Solantic include, but are not limited to, EKGs, burn treatments, hearing tests, injections, in-house lab testing such as mono, strep, urine analysis, influenza, and hemocult. These are included in the Level 2 package.

Below is a list of prices for in-patient admission testing at the primary care physician practice also in Orlando:

- Hemocult: $30
- Urine analysis: $115 (does not include cost of patient visit)
- Urine culture: $128
- Influenza: $37 for each test
- Mononucleosis: $81
- Drug Testing: $44 per test and each test includes screening for only one drug

As one can see, Solantic's services do, in fact, cost less when compared to a primary care physician practice. Based on this limited sample it would appear that services offered by retail clinics will most-likely offer consistently lower prices as compared to a physician practice.

The 2007 survey by Tu and Cohen (2008) reported that nearly all clinic users indicated that low cost was a major factor in their choice of a retail clinic rather than another venue. Moreover, retail clinics may also reduce our rapidly increasing health care costs in the United States based on our experience in markets where they have significant market penetration. An example is the Twin Cities in Minnesota, where treatment of most conditions cost twice as much in a physicians office as in a MinuteClinic (Kher, 2006).

The difference in cost has caused some insurers to provide incentives for enrollee use of clinics instead of alternatives by lowering or eliminating the co-pay. This reduces premium costs for companies represented by these insurers. The cost advantage of clinics is particularly significant and cost effective relative to emergency departments (Scott, 2006). Moreover, convenience and easy access to retail clinics may reduce employee time away from work to the benefit of employers. Convenience and affordability of clinics may also encourage care for early symptoms which may prevent longer absences from work later on (Hansen-Turton et al., 2007).

The portion of treatment cost borne by the uninsured is 100 percent. For the insured, it is usually a small co-pay. Originally retail clinics required cash payments for all services. However, now most clinic operators accept health insurance. Among the major carriers that cover services in retail clinics are United Healthcare, Aetna, CIGNA, Humana, and Medicare (Clinic Operator Web sites, 2009). Large regional health insurance carriers have also negotiated contracts with retail clinics. Most major regional and national insurers now provide coverage for clinic visits (Scott, 2007). Moreover, approximately 85% of clinics now accept insurance (Laws & Scott, 2008). As noted earlier, some larger employers now encourage clinic use for their employees by providing lower co-payments for clinic visits vs. other alternatives (Scott, 2007).

Public insurance plans have been less responsive to the growth of retail clinics. In response, many clinic providers qualified for Medicare and Medicaid reimbursement in 2007. The trend toward insurance coverage for retail clinics has not been universal. Quick-Health, for example, remains cash only since they believe most of their patients are uninsured (Tu & Cohen, 2008).

In 2007 a Harris poll indicated slightly more than 50 percent of retail clinic patients with insurance had their covered services paid by insurers (Harris Interactive, 2007). There is no question that that percentage has increased as a result of greater coverage of retail clinic services by insurers in recent years. Retail clinic patients are also more likely to use clinics as they become aware of the fact that their insurance covers clinic visits and they are required to make only small co-payments. In some cases, insurers are not requiring co-payments in order to provide incentives for consumers to utilize such clinics (*CBS News*, 2007).

A major factor in the cost advantage of retail clinics is the use of less expensive labor inputs. The major examples are nurse practitioners or physician assistants; these are obviously less costly than primary care physicians. The fact that the square footage in retail settings tends to be less than that in alternative settings also contributes to lower costs.

Quality of Care

Most health care consumers do not appear to be concerned about the staffing of retail clinics (i.e., nurse practitioners and physician assistants) or about clinical quality or safety issues. The Deloitte 2008 Survey of Health Care Consumers found the following:

- 16 percent of consumers have used a retail clinic and 34 percent indicated they were willing to do so in the future.

- 44 percent indicated they have no problems with the accuracy, safety, and quality of services provided by the nurse practitioner in a retail clinic.

- 45 percent have said they are comfortable with a nurse practitioner using computer-based systems for medical records and confirmation of treatment recommendations.

- 48 percent indicated they are comfortable with a nurse practitioner who is affiliated with a doctor's office.

- 36 percent of Medicare patients indicated they were open to using a retail clinic, and 11 percent indicated they have already done so.

- Among uninsured patients, 17 percent reported they have used retail clinics. (Deloitte Center for Health Solutions, 2008b, p. 12)

One of the reasons that patients may not be particularly concerned about safety and quality is that nurse practitioners can use computerized clinical decision support algorithms originally developed by physicians. In other words, they are providing evidence-based medicine for meeting basic primary care needs.

Retail clinics are very much aware that quality of care is a significant consumer concern. Consequently, they have focused on measuring and ensuring health care quality for consumers. While only 24 percent of clinic users believe clinics offer the same quality as other alternatives (Forrester Research, 2007), perceived quality may not have been the main driver of consumer usage. However, it is likely to be a major factor in driving future consumer demand for such services.

Clinical quality of care is now the major focus of clinic operators because they know perceived quality can make or break future demand for clinic services. MinuteClinic has already been certified by the Joint Commission (CVS Caremark Corporation, 2008). Moreover, the Continuing Care Association has voluntarily adopted ten new standards of care related to clinic relationships with local physicians, clinic relationships with other providers, technology implementation, data collection, and patient safety. Finally, several retail clinics have made a decision to use clinical guidelines recommended by the American Academy of Family Physicians (2007).

Recently, The *American Journal of Medical Quality* studied over 57,000 strep throat visits to one retail clinic to evaluate their adherence to medical guidelines related to drug therapy. Results were extremely positive with such adherence in excess of 99 percent (Woodburn, Smith, & Nelson, 2007). This study disproved the myth that clinical quality in a retail clinic may be poor and such settings may result in incentives to overprescribe medications.

The results of the study by Mundinger et al. (2007) "strongly supports the hypothesis that, using the traditional medical model of primary care, patient outcomes for NP and physician delivery of primary care do not differ" (Hansen-Turton, 2006). Therefore,

> to address the dearth of data and literature describing the full scope of services provided by nurse-managed health centers, the 2002 budget appropriation language for the Centers for Medicare and Medicaid Services (CMS) and the accompanying conference committee report included ... a demonstration project to evaluate nurse-managed health clinics in urban and rural areas across Pennsylvania, the state with the most nurse-managed clinics. (Hansen-Turton, 2006, p. 14)

In a study to evaluate the effectiveness of health clinics managed by nurses, results showed patient satisfaction with both access and the delivery process (Hansen-Turton, 2006). Moreover, patients needed fewer visits to emergency departments, shorter stays in the hospital, and fewer specialist visits. They were also less likely to have low birth weight infants relative to patients in other settings. It appears that nurse-managed health clinics are more effective in reducing the cost of care through the use of preventive health services (Convenient Care Association, 2006).

Clinical quality and assurance of such quality are crucial determinants of the long-run success of retail clinics. Retail clinic providers use standardized protocols to assist them in making clinical decisions. Such protocols are used to supplement the provider's judgment rather than replace it. The leading Continuing Care Association recommendations are based on evidence-based medicine guidelines of various physician associations (Hansen-Turton et al., 2007).

There is also a well-established process for the credentialing of nurse practitioners through their work history, which focuses on ensuring these individuals have adequate training and experience to work independently. In addition to having a Master's degree, most are certified in their specialty at the national level. Retail clinics are beginning to partner with local physicians and other health care providers through a system of mutual referrals. They also adhere to practice guidelines that exist in all states (Hansen-Turton et al., 2007).

One health care clinic called FastTrack, which is sponsored by the MeritCare Health System in Fargo, North Dakota, is described in the following case study. FastTrack is located in a grocery store, and those characteristics that enhance its quality of care for patients are described (Pollart et al., 2008).

THE FASTTRACK RETAIL CLINIC CASE

The following characteristics were described by clinic operators as quality-enhancing characteristics of their particular retail health clinic (Pollart et al., 2008):

- All of the clinic sites use the Institute for Clinical Systems Improvement clinical guidelines.
- The clinic's pediatric physician manager meets with all of the clinic's nurse practitioners to discuss department guidelines and protocols for treatment of common illnesses like middle ear infections, viral bronchitis, cold and flu symptoms, etc.
- FastTrack has also extended an invitation for physicians in the MeritCare Health System to review their clinic patient encounters and offer comments and suggestions.
- The FastTrack medical director does monthly quality monitoring of care for all patients seen in the clinic.
- The medical director can then access the records online for review.
- The clinic spends considerable time training new staff on how to readily determine if FastTrack can provide the best care possible.
- If staff determines that FastTrack is not the right place to treat a patient, he or she is quickly referred to other clinics, pediatricians, the emergency department, or his or her primary care provider.
- These patients (approximately 15 percent of patient walk-ins) are then tracked after referral to a higher level of care.
- Where appropriate, staff encourage patients to establish a medical home for ongoing or future health needs and assist them in doing so.
- Staff are respectful of established health care relationships patients may already have and will send copies of the office visit to the primary care provider upon request.

- Patient encounter records are scanned into their electronic medical record within 24–36 hours so that clinic providers and an outside primary care provider can view them.
- Staff at FastTrack are able to access the electronic records to enter immunizations, update allergies to a medication they have prescribed, and follow up on tests sent to the lab for further confirmation.
- Staff are also beginning to enter nurse practitioner care notes directly onto the electronic medical record as well as update the patient's problem and medication lists.
- New nurse practitioners for the clinic are selected based on not only their clinical skills and experience but also their ability to work autonomously, even though they are just a phone call away from support personnel within the MeritCare Health System.

While the above case study may or may not be representative of all retail clinics, it does suggest some ways in which such clinics may provide high-quality service to consumers whose needs require the limited set of services they offer. More and more such clinics are beginning to utilize these quality-enhancing techniques because they are acutely aware that their critics and consumers in general are concerned about issues in quality.

Retail clinics may also play a role in prevention and early detection of disease through immunizations and health screening. The likely result is improvements in health outcomes and quality of life related to various medical problems. In fact, the Centers for Disease Control in 2007 recognized that vaccine services at retail clinics offer an excellent way to increase adult vaccinations during influenza season. As their scale expands over time, retail clinics may be able to enhance public health surveillance and epidemiology.

Retail clinics may also be able to support aspects of disease management that is a "system of coordinated health care interventions and communications for populations with conditions in which patient self-care efforts are significant" (Lin, 2008).

Medical professionals may educate patients about disease management in terms of behavior modification, compliance, and monitoring in a retail clinic. The retail setting itself may also serve as a teaching tool. For example, a package offering of in-store nutritional tours and health monitoring services may be provided to patients with heart disease and diabetes (Lin, 2008).

Customer Satisfaction

Customer satisfaction with retail clinics is generally positive and indicates consumers are generally satisfied overall with retail clinics. A 2007 Harris poll measured customer satisfaction in the four areas of cost, convenience, qualified staff, and quality of care. Results indicated satisfaction levels between 80 and 90 percent for these four service attributes. The only surprising conclusion was that satisfaction with convenience declined from 92 percent in 2005 to 83 percent in 2007. Since convenience is a primary reason that consumers choose retail clinics (CVS Caremark Corporation, 2008) this could be an impediment to future growth of clinics.

Table 6.2 reports on customer satisfaction of a national sample of 2,441 adults with retail health care clinic experience in 2007. Fifty-two percent were very satisfied with the clinical quality of services provided and another 38 perent were somewhat satisfied. Similar very high percentages, ranging from 84 to 90 percent, were very satisfied or somewhat satisfied with cost, convenience, and staff qualifications in retail clinics. The percentage of dissatisfied customers for each service attribute was very low, ranging from 3 to

TABLE 6.2 Consumer Satisfaction with Retail Health Clinics by Service Attribute, 2007

Service Attributes	Very Satisfied (%)	Somewhat Satisfied (%)	Not at All/ Not Very Satisfied (%)	Not Sure (%)
Quality of Care	52	38	3	7
Cost	52	28	8	12
Convenience	63	21	4	13
Qualified Staff	53	32	4	11

Note: Percentages may not add up to 100 percent due to rounding. Results represent online survey of 2,441 U.S. adults ages 18 and older conducted by Harris Interactive between March 20 and 22, 2007.

Source: Harris Interactive. (2007, April 11). "Most Adults Satisfied with Care at Retail Based Health Clinics." *Health Care Poll, 6*(6).

8 percent. Similarly, Walmart has found customer satisfaction in its clinics to be over 90 percent in terms of overall customer satisfaction with their total experience (Walmart, 2006).

In the previously discussed demonstration project looking at evaluating nurse-managed clinics, results indicated patients were very satisfied with clinic access and the process of service delivery (Hansen-Turton et al., 2004). This result is consistent with previous research showing that patients consistently rate their satisfaction with care provided by nurse practitioners as very high (Hansen-Turton, 2007).

The case study reported in the previous section by Pollart et al. (2008) also shows that patient satisfaction is extremely high at the FastTrack clinic in Fargo, North Dakota. They report that customers love the convenience. Below are a couple of quotes from their customers:

> I was there the Saturday before Christmas, so a very busy day. I needed to get groceries before we left town, and my ears were bothering me . . . stopped at FastTrack, saw the NP and was on my way in a few minutes. Very quick. Where else can you get your ears checked, buy groceries, and get a latte all at the same time.
>
> I had been dragging with a cold for a couple of weeks, and my ear was bothering me. Within fifteen minutes, I was seen, a diagnosis was made, a prescription was given, my insurance form submitted, I paid the bill and was on-time for my next business appointment. And much to my amazement, I received a hand-written thank you note from the provider a few days later. I was appreciated as a customer! This is how I want my healthcare delivered: efficient, effective, and friendly.

Negative feedback at FastTrack has been minimal. The few complaints received had to do with insurance filing and one other due to a long wait when the clinic was inundated with sports physicals.

In sum, patient satisfaction has been extremely high at FastTrack and most patients become "raving fans." Patients have no quality concerns and actually prefer to be seen by the nurse practitioner for minor ailments. This may force other primary care delivery sites to improve their service delivery systems to be more convenient and cost effective.

Although the majority of consumers are pleased with their physician providers, hospitals, and other primary care health care providers, they do want better service and improved value. The Deloitte 2008 Survey of Health Care Consumers indicated somewhat lower ratings for primary care physicians than for retail clinics, as follows:

- Primary care physicians showed average satisfaction ratings of 82 where 0 equals completely dissatisfied and 100 equals completely satisfied.
- Almost a third of the respondents indicated a desire for service improvements such as more physician face time, shorter waits for service, and more rapid appointments. At this point in time, it appears that retail clinics may provide somewhat higher levels of customer satisfaction than do other primary care service providers due to their accessibility, convenience, and low cost. Apparently, quality of care is not a factor that has detracted from customer satisfaction with retail clinics in the provision of such services.

Transparency/Accountability

Retail clinics have led the way in providing the consumer with complete pricing transparency by providing a full menu of their available services with all prices clearly displayed. As a result, consumers know their costs prior to receiving services.

By comparison, most other health care service providers have been less transparent and accountable to the customer for the cost of the services they provide. The consumer has been shielded from the actual cost of the services they are receiving. As a result, consumers have not been effective in forcing providers to become more efficient in ways that reduce costs and improve quality simultaneously.

The retail clinics at Walmart emphasize the fact that they provide everyday low prices for routine "get well" visits to one of their clinics, which typically cost between $40 and $65. They emphasize price transparency as a major marketing approach as evidenced by prominent price lists that let patients know in advance what their charges will be. "Knowing exactly how much services are going to cost matters a whole lot more to customers who have to pay all cost out of pocket . . . sometimes you have $39, but you don't have $149. If you are low income and you are going to get a bill, you have to think about it" (Walmart, 2006).

Coordination of Care

One of the issues raised by critics of retail health care clinics is that they may contribute to further fragmentation of the patient care processes. This would be particularly true if clinics were unable or unwilling to communicate and coordinate their patient care services with other providers (Bodenheimer, 2008). Most retail health clinic providers today can and do use their electronic medical records to furnish a patient visit summary and fax that summary and the electronic medical record to any other provider upon the patient's request. However, there are no data indicating to what degree such communication has actually occurred and whether it is greater than communication between traditional providers (Bodenheimer, 2008).

Most clinics will refer those patients needing services not provided by the clinic to other primary or specialist providers in the community. Most clinics are able to share patient records electronically with those providers who are able to process them (Hansen-Turton, 2007). Even when the primary care physician does not have an electronic medical record system, the clinic may provide a printed record that the patient may share with his primary care physician. The result is a higher level of continuity of care that should enhance the long-term health status of patients. Consequently, retail clinics can and do coordinate their care with such providers if such coordination is desired by the patient.

Coordination of care for those with chronic conditions is particularly relevant in this respect. Asheville, North Carolina, has partnered with local retail clinic pharmacists to significantly reduce its costs for employees with diabetes. These pharmacists conduct routine exams on a regular basis and send patients who need intervention immediately to their providers (Turner, 2007). Employees are also rewarded with free medications for keeping their appointments.

Walmart now operates some of its in-store health clinics in partnership with local hospitals under "The Clinic at Walmart" brand. Previously, Walmart had partnered with retail clinic providers to provide all of its retail clinic services. The new co-branded clinics are now available in many cities. The advantage to Walmart is that their clinics are integrated with well-known and well-respected health care provider systems in the community.

Another example related to Walmart is a partnership between the company and two clinic providers to run telemedicine clinics in a few Houston-area stores. One of the companies (NuPhysicia) operates the largest and oldest telemedicine program in the United States. The clinic company, My Healthy Access, operates the clinics. The telemedicine component allows external physicians to communicate directly with clinic staff in real time. These physicians can guide the staff member who is actually providing the care to the patient (Walmart Stores, 2009).

Finally, Cleveland Clinic recently partnered with MinuteClinic in several Ohio CVS retail clinics. Nine locations are staffed by nurse practitioners supported by an on-site medical director from the Cleveland Clinic. The goal is to provide continuity of care between the CVS retail clinics and the Cleveland Clinic. It has been an innovative solution that addresses consumers' desires for access, affordability, and quality of primary health care services as well as coordination of all levels of care across different providers ("Cleveland Clinic Teams with MinuteClinic," 2009).

Financial Viability

Retail clinics are able to provide their services at lower costs through the use of less expensive labor as noted earlier. The fact that they are exempt from certain hygiene requirements and provide services with minimal square footage enhances their cost advantage relative to alternatives (Deloitte Center for Health Solutions, 2008a).

Despite these cost advantages, profitability and financial viability of clinics require a high volume of services. The average 450-square-foot retail clinic costs have been estimated at $600,000/year (California HealthCare Foundation, 2006). Since the typical retail clinic service cost about $60 in 2006, an annual volume of 10,000 patients plus would be required to cover its costs. However, a break-even point would also have to cover all of the variable costs of providing these services. Consequently, retail clinics would need about 12,000 plus patient visits per year to cover both fixed and variable costs and earn a profit (California HealthCare Foundation, 2006). In 2010 these numbers would need to be adjusted upward.

The financial status of retail clinics is not well known because details are scarce. There may be approximately 1,100 retail clinics in the United States in 2010. It was previously estimated that there are 115 million low acuity and nonurgent primary care visits per year (Deloitte, 2008a). If the break-even point for the average clinic is 11,000 visits per year, total annual patient visits per year would need to exceed 9 million visits a year for the overall retail clinic industry to be profitable. This would be between 7–8 percent of overall demand for low acuity and non-urgent conditions. Although volume is moving in the right direction, we have not yet achieved that volume of retail clinic visits as of 2010 (Deloitte Center for Health Solutions, 2008a).

In addition to the concerns mentioned above, Dr. William Winkenwerder has noted a couple of other concerns regarding the future financial viability of retail clinics as follows:

- First is the potential for significant medical liability cases with associated expenses and adverse publicity. Trial attorneys will find the deep pockets of large corporations that operate retail clinics even more appealing than that of practicing physicians. I offer these cautions: Watch out! You are operating in a target-rich environment. Providing consistently high-quality medical care is never as easy as it looks. Also, mitigate your risks by using evidence-based protocols, seek appropriate accreditation and find a group of expert medical advisors to guide your ongoing efforts.
- The second risk to the future of retail medical clinics is the prospect of efforts to regulate clinics to the point where they are not economically viable. Physician organizations will be the main protagonists, but state and federal lawmakers will be the ultimate determinants, as they must balance the obvious public needs that can be met with retail clinics with reasonable assurances of proper operation and oversight. On a personal level, having practiced for years with nurse practitioners and physician assistants, I believe firmly that such professionals can offer excellent medical care. (2009)

In sum, it appears that despite the success of retail clinics in terms of enhancing access, mitigating concerns about quality, enhancing convenience, and reducing costs for certain services, the jury is still out regarding their present and future financial viability. If these clinics are able to build their volume to a greater degree than they have thus far (2010), then their financial future may be quite bright. In addition, if one were to consider cross-selling to consumers beyond the profit and loss of the clinics themselves, then some clinics that may appear unprofitable in terms of their direct revenues and costs may be profitable and worth maintaining due to other consumer purchases at the time they received service in a retail health clinic.

CONCLUSION

It appears that retail clinics are serving both an underserved segment of our population (i.e., those who are uninsured or underinsured, low income families, young people, families with children) as well as insured individuals and families who seek primary health care services in a more convenient setting with longer hours, geographic proximity, and no need for appointments. As such, retail clinics fill a market niche that had not been previously well served by other primary care service health care providers.

Performance of retail health clinics is generally good for the range of services they provide. Moreover, they may be more advanced and more sophisticated in the use of technology for patient records and protocols for patient care than are primary physician offices. They appear to excel in terms of access, convenience, and low costs vis-à-vis primary care providers. In addition, their quality of care appears to be at least equal to the quality of care provided in other settings.

What is still uncertain is their financial long-term viability. In many retail settings, and for many service providers, retail clinics are still in a "start-up" stage. This means that they have not yet attained their projected patient volumes and revenues. Many are losing money because the patient volumes do not yet cover fixed costs.

The question for the future is to what degree volumes will grow. This is a function of many variables, including their ability to modify their clinic models to better fit the varying consumer markets in which they operate, economic conditions that allow families to self-fund their care at such clinics or mostly pay for their care through their health insurance, and government regulation that may encourage or discourage future clinic growth in various parts of the country. The latter will be discussed in the next chapter.

REFERENCES

Agency for Healthcare Research and Quality. (2006). *Consumer assessment of health plan satisfaction.* https://www.cahps.ahrq.gov/content/ncbd/Chartbook/2006_CAHPS_HealthPlanChartbook.pdf.

American Academy of Family Physicians. (2007). http://www.aafp.org/online/en/home/media/releases/2007/20070201clinicattributes.html.

BMC Health Services Research. (2007). http://www.pubmedcentral.nih.gov/picrender.fcgi?artid=1810532&blobtype=pdf.

Bodenheimer, T. 2008., "Coordinating care—A perilous journey through the health care system," *New England Journal of Medicine, 358*(10), 1064–1071.

California HealthCare Foundation. (2006). http://www.chcf.org/topics/view.cfm?itemID=123218.

CBS News. (2007). http://www.cbsnews.com/stories/2007/08/11/health/main3158978.shtml.

Centers for Disease Control. (2007). *Strategies for increasing adult vaccination rates.* Atlanta, GA: Centers for Disease Control.

Centers for Disease Control and Prevention. (2006). *National hospital ambulatory medical care survey: 2004 emergency department summary.* http://www.cdc.gov/nchs/data/ad/ad372.pdf.

"Cleveland Clinic teams with MinuteClinic." (2007). Accessed at http://www.immediatecarebusiness.com/hotnews/cleveland-clinic–minuteclinic-team-up.html.

Clinic operator Web sites. (2009). http://minuteclinic.com/en/USA/Treatment-and-Cost.aspx; http://takecarehealth.com; http://www.rediclinic.com/services/services.asp.

Convenient Care Association. (2006). Nurse practitioners: Providing cost-effective, quality care when you need it most." Convenient Care Association Web site. Available at http://www.ccaclinics.org.

CVS Caremark Corporation. (2008). http://investor.cvs.com/phoenix.zhtml?c=99533&p=irol-newsArticle&ID=907392.

Deloitte Center for Health Solutions. (2008a). *Retail clinics: Facts, trends, and implications.* Accessed May 19, 2009, at http://www.deloitte.com/centerforhealthsolutions.

Deloitte Center for Health Solutions. (2008b). *2008 Survey of health care consumers: Executive summary.* Accessed May 20, 2009, at http://www.deloitte.com/centerforhealthsolutions.

Deloitte Center for Health Solutions. (2008c). *Growth of retail clinics: 2008 Survey of health care consumers.* Accessed May 19, 2009, from http://www.deloitte.com/dtt/article/0,1002,sid%253D127087%2526cid%253D192463,00.html.

Druss, B. G., Marcus, S. C., Olfson, M., Tanielien, M., & Pincus, H. A. (2003). Trends in care by nonphysician clinicians in the United States. *New England Journal of Medicine, 348,* 130–137.

Forrester Research. (2007). *Retail health clinics: Convenience trumps service and quality.* http://www.forrester.com/Research/Document/0,7211,41216,00.html.

Green, L., Dodoo, M., Ruddy, G., et al. (2004). *The physician workforce of the United States: A family medicine perspective.* The Robert Graham Center Web site. Available at http://www.graham-center.org/online/graham/home.html (accessed October 10, 2006).

Hansen-Turton, T. (2006). *The nurse-managed health center safety net: A policy solution to reducing health disparities,* 1st ed. New York: Elsevier–Saunders.

Hansen-Turton, T., Line, L., O'Connell, M., Rothman, N., & Lauby, J. (2004). Report to the Centers for Medicare and Medicaid Services: The nursing model of health care for the underserved. Available at www.nncc.us/programs/CMS%20Revised-Section1(CovTitleAck)-Submitted120604.doc.

Hansen-Turton, T., Ryan, S., Miller, K., Counts, M., & Nash, D. B. (2007). Convenient care clinics: The future of accessible health care. *Disease Management, 10*(2), 61–73.

Harris Interactive. (2005). *Many agree on potential benefits of onsite clinics in major retail stores that can provide basic medical services, yet large numbers are also skeptical.* http://www.harrisinteractive.com/news/allnewsbydate.asp?NewsID=983.

Harris Interactive. (2007). *Most adults satisfied with care at retail-based health clinics.* http://www.harrisinteractive.com/news/allnewsbydate.asp?NewsID=1201.

Henry J. Kaiser Family Foundation. 2006. "The uninsured: A primer, key facts about americans without health insurance."

Herzlinger, R. (2007). Who killed U.S. medicine? *The Washington Post*, p. A15. Retrieved from http://www.washingtonpost.com/wp-dyn/content/article/2007/07/24/AR2007072401850.html.

Kennedy, J., et al. (2004). Access to emergency care: restricted by long waiting times and cost and coverage concerns. *Annals of Emergency Medicine, 43*(5), 567–573.

Kher, U. (2006, March 20). Get a check-up in aisle three." *Time*, 52–53.

Lando, L. (2006, July 20). The new force in walk-in clinics. *Wall Street Journal*, D1, D2.

Laws, M., and Scott, M. K. (2008). The emergence of retail-based clinics in the United States: Early observations. *Health Affairs, 27*(5), 1293–1298.

Lin, D. Q. (2008). Convenience care clinics: Opposition, opportunity, and the path to health system integration. *Frontiers of Health Services Management, 24*(3), 3–11.

Mehrotra, A., Wang, M. C., Lave, J. R., Adams, J. L., & McGlynn, E. A. (2008). Retail clinics, primary care physicians, and emergency departments: A comparison of physician business. *Health Affairs, 27*(5), 1275–1282.

Mundinger, M. O., Kane, R. L., Lenz, E. R., et al. (2000). Primary care outcomes in patients treated by nurse practitioners or physicians. *JAMA, 283*, 59.

Murray, M., & Berwick, D. M. (2003). Advanced access: Reducing waiting and delays in primary care. *Journal of the American Medical Association, 289*(8), 1035–1049.

Pollert, P., Dobberstein, D., & Wiisanen, R. (2008). Jumping into the healthcare retail market: Our experience. *Frontiers of Health Services Management, 24*(3), 13–21. Retrieved from Business Source Premier database.

Scott, M. K. (2006). Health care in the express lane: The emergence of retail clinics. California HealthCare Foundation Web site. http://www.chcf.org/topics/view.cfm?itemID=123218 (accessed October 10, 2006).

Scott, M. K. (2007). Health care in the express lane: Retail clinics go main-stream. Report to the California HealthCare Foundation.

Tu, H. T., & Cohen, G. R. (2008, December). *Checking up on retail based health clinics: Is the boom ending?* The Commonwealth Fund. Issues Brief No. 1199. New York: The Commonwealth Fund.

Turner, G. M. (2007, May 14). Customer health care. *Wall Street Journal*, A17.

Walmart Stores. (2006). *"The Clinic at Walmart" to open in Atlanta, Little Rock and Dallas Supercenters.* http://walmartfacts.com/_resources/ToolBar/printerfriendly.aspx?id=5651&pagetyp (accessed February 11, 2008).

Walmart Stores. (2009). *Two companies to run Walmart telemedicine clinics.* http://walmartfacts.com/_resources/ToolBar/printerfriendly.aspx?id=192014&pagetyp (accessed March 15, 2009).

Winkenwerder, W. (2009). *Retail medical clinics: Here to stay?* http://www.deloitte.com/dtt/article/0,1002,sid%253D127087%2526cid%253D192739,00.html (accessed May 20, 2009).

Woodburn, J. D., Smith, K. L., & Nelson, G. D. (2007). Quality of care in the retail health care setting using national clinical guidelines for acute pharyngitis. *American Journal of Medical Quality, 22*(6), 457–462.

Chapter 7

The Impact of Retail Clinics on Other Stakeholders

In this chapter, we will address major winners and losers among all stakeholders impacted by the introduction and growth of retail health clinics. First we will consider the impact of retail health clinics on other health care providers. Then we will consider their impact on other nonprovider stakeholders such as patients, health plans, employers, and public officials/policy makers.

MAJOR WINNERS AND LOSERS AMONG HEALTH CARE PROVIDERS

Table 7.1 offers a stakeholder assessment that describes the potential benefits and disadvantages that retail clinics offer for a variety of health care providers. Based on this assessment, potential winners and losers are identified.

Primary Care Physicians

In the future, physicians may become more competitive with retail clinics in terms of convenience. For example, they could extend their hours to evenings and weekends. However, lowering their prices to become cost competitive with retail clinics will be more difficult. In any economy, services that can be provided more economically will be provided more economically. Since physicians are not likely to be competitive with retail clinics in terms of their pricing, insurers will likely begin to shift more coverage of enrollee minor health conditions from physicians to retail clinics.

TABLE 7.1 Major Winners and Losers Among Health Care Providers

Stakeholder	Potential Benefits	Potential Disadvantages	Winner/Loser/Neutral—Why?
Physicians— Primary Care	Reduce physician's crowded waiting rooms as well as working late hours to accommodate "unscheduled patients" with basic care needs such as earaches and colds.	Could experience significant financial losses as clinics acquire a lucrative segment of the practice—basic or routine medical care (particularly if health clinics include them in network). May be unable to sustain private practice without this segment.	Loser: Less expensive substitutes (NPs, PAs, etc.) will perform much of the routine care previously provided by the primary care physician. Could mitigate loss through formal collaboration with clinics.
Physicians— Specialists	Referrals for more specialized care may come from these clinics.	Could face competition from primary care physicians who might shift into one or more specialties.	Winner: Potential for referrals from retail clinics.
Medical Groups (not affiliated with hospitals)	Become more efficient in order to compete with retail clinics. Become truly customer focused to ensure repeat business.	May lose ground to retail clinics because of loss of profitable patients with minor conditions as well as the clinics' expanded hours of operation, convenience, and low cost. May be left with low margin, chronically ill patients.	Loser: May eventually recede from the health care landscape much as the "Mom & Pop" retail stores, supermarkets, and pharmacies have declined in the face of competition from "big box" retailers.

Nurses (NPs, APNs, etc.) and Physician Assistants (PAs)	Retail clinics represent an additional option of employment for these advanced degreed clinicians. Technology will enable these practitioners to use their education and training to provide basic care needs for patients and in some states to write prescriptions.	May be viewed by some physicians (primary care) as competitors. There may be some legislative efforts by physician organizations to restrict professional practice acts for these professions.	Winner: Increased professional opportunities as well as job autonomy.
Hospitals and Health Systems • Nonprofit • For profit • Academic Health Center	Allow hospitals or systems to focus on their core business, and match resources to skill level required to attend to patients with basic care needs.	Potential to suffer reduced revenue generation from EDs and ambulatory clinics. New network relationships with clinics might cause friction with physician network.	Winner/Loser? This will depend on how much of their revenue derives from providing basic medical care. Potential to win if hospitals collaborate with, become subcontractors for, and extend services of retail clinics.

Urgent Care Clinics	Reduce overcrowded waiting rooms—similar to EDs (see below).	Because these clinics also tend to see patients with routine or basic care needs, there is the potential to gain revenue as complements to retail clinics.	Winner: Patients tend to go to these clinics because they have nowhere else to go—even if the care they seek is routine care. Retail clinics will attract patients seeking routine care because of affordability and convenience. Patients with urgent care needs, who could not be accommodated in overcrowded EDs, may find increased access in less crowded urgent care clinics.
Emergency Departments (EDs)	Reduce the number of patients seeking emergency care for nonemergent medical needs by offering an alternative.	May lose patient revenue to retail clinics. Patients with emergency conditions may self-refer to the retail clinic. The clinic will then have to refer them to the ED, adding another step in the process and wasting time.	Winner: Potential to reduce some overcrowding, especially nonemergent cases. However, this may also be associated with a loss of revenue.

If insurers decide that primary care physicians are too expensive in providing routine or basic care, these physicians may be among the biggest losers (Malvey & Fottler, 2006).

Various physician associations have responded to the growth of retail clinics by advocating various impediments and increased regulation of the industry. They have also advocated various clinical guidelines to address alleged quality of care concerns. In response, the retail clinic industry has offered to work in collaboration with physicians to enhance both access and quality of patients for primary care services.

The American Academy of Family Physicians (AAFP) spoke out publicly in 2006 about their view of retail clinics (AAFP, 2006). After studying the growth and evolution of retail clinics in the United States, the AAFP made a decision to attempt to shape the model of care in retail clinics in order to benefit patients. Toward that end, the AAFP developed a list of desirable clinic attributes in order to enhance patient safety and quality of care:

- Retail clinics must have a well-defined and clinical scope of services.
- Clinical services and treatment must be evidence-based and quality improvement oriented.
- The clinic should have a formal connection with physician practices in the local community to provide continuity of care.
- Other health professionals, such as nurse practitioners, should only operate in accordance with state and local regulations, as part of a "team-based" approach and under responsible supervision of a practicing, licensed physician.
- The clinic should have a referral system to physician practices or other entities appropriate to the patients' symptoms beyond the clinic's scope of work.
- The clinic should encourage all patients to have a "medical home."
- The clinic should include an electronic health records system sufficient to gather and communicate the patient's information to the family physician's office, preferably one that is compatible with the Continuity of Care Record supported by AAFP and others.

More recently, the AAFP has met with leaders of some of the major clinic companies such as MinuteClinic, Take Care, and Redi-Clinic. As a result, these companies have expressed support for the AAFP's desired attributes. Recently the American Medical Association (AMA) has also proposed retail clinic guidelines that are quite similar to the AAFP desired attributes.

Some are concerned that as more primary care services shift to retail clinics, this could negatively impact primary care physicians (Bohmer, 2007). Farber, Siu, and Bloom (2007) found that the visits for the most common patient complaints addressed by retail clinics require approximately 25 percent less time than other patient visits. Consequently, if more patients shift to retail clinics, primary care physicians will need to schedule fewer patients per hour. It is quite possible that a shift in patients to retail clinics could hurt primary care physicians financially.

However, these physicians could replace the basic primary care visits with visits addressing more complex problems. The result would be higher reimbursement so that the lower patient volume would be offset by higher reimbursement for the remaining patients. Obviously, this is a questions that needs to be researched in the future.

Several retail clinic companies are partnering or attempting to partner with the medical and nursing communities in their areas. The basic purpose is to determine how they might work together to serve the needs of patients in terms of access, quality, and integration of services (Hansen-Turton et al., 2007). The increase in demand for services in retail clinics results from the current limitations on access to care for many patients (American Academy of Pediatrics, 2006). In the future, continued dialog between retail clinics and local medical and nursing practitioners is critical to enhance patient care.

Retail clinics have been the subject of controversy from their very beginnings in 2000. A number of physician associations have raised concerns about the quality of care in such settings in terms of potential inaccurate diagnoses, inappropriate triage decisions, and a lack of communication with existing physician providers. In addition to the American Medical Association, other associations of primary care physicians (Family Physicians and Pediatricians) have also raised concerns (Japsen, 2007; Retail-Based Clinical Policy Workgroup, 2006; American Academy of Family Physicians, 2007).

However, advocates for retail clinics argue that quality and safety concerns raised by physician groups are not valid and are actually motivated by the financial concerns of physicians (Seward, 2007). They note that primary care physicians are likely to lose some business if patients with minor ailments choose to address their concerns at a retail clinic instead of a physician office.

Table 7.2 summarizes the quality standards developed by the Convenient Care Association (CCA) in response to all of the criticisms coming from the medical community. This association attempts to provide consumers with accessible, affordable, quality health care in retail-based locations through the sharing of best practices and common standards of operation. They also strive to enhance and sustain the growth of the Convenient Care industry, which was founded in October 2006.

Specialist Physicians

Many of the concerns expressed in the previous section might also apply to specialist physicians although to a lesser degree. Currently, these physicians are not in direct competition with retail clinics and, therefore, are not likely to suffer a revenue loss as a result. In addition, they may be able and willing to formally collaborate with such clinics so that patients who present themselves with symptoms relevant to that specialty may be referred to these specialist physicians. Obviously, this would enhance their referral base and their revenues. The only potential downside is that some primary care physicians may begin to practice in certain specialties as their revenue base is eroded as a result of retail clinics.

Medical Practices

Only about 10 percent of retail clinic visits result in a referral of the patient to an alternative setting. As a result, retail clinics appear to be attracting patients away from other alternative primary care settings. Consequently, these providers are likely to experience some significant decline in demand for their services. While these traditional primary care providers will continue to dominate those certain services not offered by retail clinics, the latter are likely to dominate overlapping services. The only potential impediment to such domination would be patient concerns about quality of care.

In response to the competitive threat of retail clinics, some physicians now offer more flexible hours and a greater emphasis on serving the customer. If retail clinics begin to offer care for more acute and chronic conditions, medical groups will undoubtedly become more adversarial since they would be competing for the same base of patients.

The future potential growth of retail clinics is also clouded by a potential negative reaction from physicians and physician groups.

TABLE 7.2　Quality of Care Standards of the Convenient Care Association of America

- All providers will be thoroughly credentialed for license, training, and experience, with rigorous background checks to verify training and licensing.
- All CCA Members are committed to monitoring quality on an ongoing basis, including but not limited to:
  - peer review;
  - collaborating physician review;
  - use of evidence-based guidelines;
  - collecting aggregate data on selected quality and safety outcomes;
  - collecting patient satisfaction data.

- All CCA Members build relationships with traditional health care providers and hospitals, and work towards a goal of using EHRs to share patient information and ensure continuity of care.
- All CCA Members are committed to encouraging patients to establish a relationship with a primary care provider, and to making appropriate and careful referrals for follow-on care and for conditions that are outside of the scope of the clinic's services.
- All CCA Members are in compliance with applicable OSHA, CLIA, HIPAA, and ADA standards. All CCA Members follow Centers for Disease Control (CDC) guidelines for infection control through hand washing.
- All CCA Members provide health promotion and disease prevention education to patients. All CCA Members provide written instructions and educational materials to patients upon leaving the clinic.
- All CCA Members use Electronic Health Records (EHR) to ensure high-quality efficient care. All CCA Members are committed to providing all patients with the opportunity to share health information with other providers electronically or in paper format.
- All CCA Members provide an environment conducive to quality patient care and meet standards for infection control and safety.
- All CCA Members will establish emergency response procedures and develop relationships with local emergency response service providers to ensure that patients in need of emergency care can be transported to an appropriate setting as quickly as possible.
- CCA Members empower patients to make informed choices about their health care. Prices for services provided at Convenient Care Clinics are readily available in a visible place outside of the examination room. Providers discuss what impact, if any, the provision of additional services will have on the ultimate cost of the patient.

Source: Convenient Care Association Quality and Safety Standards, http://www.ccaclinics.org/index.php?option=com_content&view=article&id=6:quality-of-care&catid=3:about-us&Itemid=13

Physicians may pressure their legislators to restrict retail clinics and make them unprofitable. Alternatively they may choose to compete through the extension of their office hours or the provision of same-day scheduling (Bachman, 2006). The latter response may result in patients experiencing improved access to their regular providers as well as weaker incentives to opt for retail clinics as a source for routine primary care services.

Retail clinics and physicians throughout the United States have collaborated and partnered in developing mutually beneficial relationships to serve their patient populations. Some physicians welcome retail clinics as a good primary care alternative for their patients while others oppose the formation of retail clinics. The latter base their opposition on potential lack of quality care, assessments that nurse practitioners are not qualified to work independently and that the patients would not receive integrated care. Many physicians today recognize that retail clinics provide a needed alternative for certain services for their patients that are not provided by traditional providers (Hansen-Turton et al., 2007).

Nurses and Physician Assistants

Nurses and physician assistants are likely winners as they gain opportunities to practice outside of the physician's office or hospital. Obviously, retail clinics offer increased employment opportunities for both nurse practitioners and physician assistants. In some states, their scope of practice may increase when they are employed in retail clinics; however, primary care physicians may pressure regulators in some states to restrict the practice of nurse practitioners and physician assistants in order to reduce competition.

Hospitals and Health Systems

Hospital emergency departments are also expected to be winners. Emergency care nationwide is in crisis because of overcrowding, partly because patients are using the emergency department for nonemergencies. For example, the Florida Hospital Association (FHA) recently reported that patients are going to the emergency department because they are open evenings and weekend hours, they do not need an appointment, and they lack access to other nonemergency services (FHA, 2005). In addition, hospitals have the potential to be winners, particularly if they become subcontractors for retail health clinics (Malvey & Fottler, 2006).

Many health systems are now operating retail clinics to exploit the increased popularity of retail settings. One example is Mayo Clinic, which has opened retail clinics in Minnesota to compete with MinuteClinic, which has grown rapidly in that state. Other examples include Sutter Express Care in Northern California, Geisinger Careworks in Central Pennsylvania, AtlantiCare HealthRite in New Jersey, and Aurora QuickCare in Wisconsin (Deloitte Center for Health Solutions, 2008).

Most integrated health systems in the United States have a recognizable brand that is recognized in their own communities. This should provide them some competitive advantage in competing with other retail clinic operators. These systems are becoming more adept at establishing clinics in their local communities. For example AtlantiCare has developed a turnkey model and is currently using that model to assist other health systems to establish their own retail health clinics (Finarelli & Pillai, 2007; *Journal of Healthcare Contracting*, 2007).

Since local and regional health systems are well known in their own communities, they may be better positioned than retailers and retail clinic companies to attract local patients to retail clinics. For example, they would not have to market as intensively due to their high visibility. Other health systems are choosing a different model by forming partnerships with other large retailers to open co-branded clinics (Armstrong, 2008).

Urgent Care Clinics

Urgent care centers are expected to be among the winners because they provide acute care in a less-expensive setting than physician offices and EDs. Moreover, in many instances, urgent care centers are open for extended hours. For example, in Florida, about 25 percent of urgent care centers are open past 8:00 PM (FHA, 2005).

Both physician offices and urgent care clinics are currently attempting to become more customer service oriented and attempting to differentiate their services in terms of high-quality care. Finally, electronic medical records are now being provided on the Web and most providers now provide electronic prescribing for their patients.

Emergency Departments

Hospital emergency departments are also expected to be winners. Emergency care nationwide is in crisis because of overcrowding, partly because patients are using the emergency department for nonemergencies. Retail clinics may help to alleviate some of that overcrowding. In addition, hospitals have the potential to be winners, particularly if they become subcontractors for retail health clinics.

MAJOR WINNERS AND LOSERS AMONG OTHER STAKEHOLDERS

Table 7.3 outlines the major winners and losers among other stakeholders who are not direct providers of services to health care consumers. Among these are patients, health plans, employers, and public officials/policy makers.

Patients

Patients are obvious winners with retail health clinics because they offer greater geographical access, greater access in terms of hours of operation, and lower out-of-pocket expenses to the consumer. The fact that no appointments are required is another obvious benefit. These benefits have been outlined in some detail in Chapters 5 and 6.

Retail clinics offer particular benefits to patients who lack a primary care physician, including young people, minorities, and low income groups. The only potential disadvantage for patients is that some may fail to seek out a "medical home" or a primary care physician.

Health Plans

Insurers and other third-party payers are expected to become winners because the retail health care costs are much lower than traditional settings, especially emergency departments. They now realize that encouraging enrollees to use retail clinics as an alternative to other settings can create cost savings. As a result, some insurers no longer require co-payments as they encourage patients to choose retail clinics over other primary care settings. One Minnesota insurer (HealthPartners) found that a patient visit was, on

TABLE 7.3   Major Winners and Losers Among Other Stakeholders

Stakeholder	Potential Benefits	Potential Disadvantages	Winner/Loser/ Neutral—Why?
Patients	Easier access to and lower costs for basic services.	May not seek a "medical home."	Winner: Greater access to basic services at a lower cost.
Health Plans	Payers may end up paying less for basic care for patients. Enrollee satisfaction might increase with inclusion of clinics in network.	Discount retailers may end up as competitors by offering insurance products of their own (i.e., Costco).	Winner: Will save money because the retail clinics' charges reflect the use of technology and less skilled personnel to perform basic care.
Employers	Reduced absenteeism and emergency department use. Could reduce costs through retail clinics and their potential for disease management and occupational health programs.	Serious employee health problems may not be diagnosed early, thus leading to higher long-term costs.	Winner: Easier access for employees together with lower insurance costs and prevention options.
Public Officials/Policy Makers	Greater access for underserved groups. Lower costs for basic services.	Could suffer criticism from certain constituencies due to inadequate regulation.	Winner: Greater access at lower costs for consumers.

average, $18 cheaper in a retail clinic than in other, traditional primary care settings (Schmit, 2006).

It is possible that if insurers waive co-pays and allow patients to receive service in convenient retail clinics, the cost savings may be offset by higher consumer use of this low-cost care. Obviously, they do not wish to increase the probability that enrollees seek unnecessary care and add to the insurers' costs. In the long run, however, health plans might benefit financially if they were to partner with retail clinics to offer enhanced preventive care. This might lower the long-term costs of more acute illnesses treated in nonprimary care settings.

As noted above, health insurers have seen significant cost savings when their enrollees use retail clinics. While a primary care physician visit typically costs an insurer about $110, the same service provided in a retail clinic may cost $60 or less. These savings are particularly significant in the case of a hospital emergency department (Spencer, 2005).

Some insurers lower the patient co-pay in order to create incentives for patients to use clinics in preference to other alternatives. Blue Cross Blue Shield of Minnesota has already altered co-pays so that enrollees pay little or nothing if they choose a retail clinic over a physician office visit. Several health insurers in Portland, Oregon, offer similar incentives (Spencer, 2005).

Employers

Employers need to attract and retain high-quality labor in order to remain competitive in their markets. To do so they must offer cost-effective benefits that these employees value. As a result, many employers are receptive to retail clinics if they become convinced such clinics offer quality care for lower costs. Employers can achieve significant cost savings when they design benefit packages that encourage employees to choose retail clinics over more expensive primary care settings (Deloitte Center for Health Solutions, 2008).

The convenient location of retail clinics might also enhance employee health and productivity. Instead of taking time off to visit more traditional providers, employees could plan to visit a retail clinic while traveling to and from work or during various breaks during the day. Likewise, parents could take their children to a retail clinic instead of waiting for an appointment with their pediatrician. As a result, attendance might increase and tardiness might be reduced to the benefit of both employer and employee.

Employer health insurance costs might also be reduced as a result of less use of hospital emergency departments. Employee wellness initiatives, disease management services, and occupational health services could also be provided though contracts with retail clinics.

Recently, many small companies have begun to drop health care insurance coverage for their employees as a result of the recession (Mattioli, 2009). One way small companies may avoid dropping health insurance coverage might be to encourage their employees to seek out primary care services at retail clinics. Even if they do end up dropping health insurance, they might write a contract with local retail clinics to provide basic services for their employees at the employers' expense.

Public Officials/Policy Makers

Policy makers at the federal, state, and local levels face continually tighter budgets as they attempt to provide accessible and quality services for their constituents while trying to contain health care costs. The fiscal crisis has exacerbated this challenge (Deloitte Center for Health Solutions, 2008).

They could partner with retail clinics to monitor and measure sentinel health events and prepare their constituents for possible future pandemics. Policy makers could also support the growth of retail clinics by allowing an expansion in the nurse practitioner's scope of practice as well as liability protection for retail clinic medical directors. Such initiatives could facilitate the expansion of retail clinics to lower income communities.

One of the major factors driving the existence or growth of retail clinics is the regulatory climate in each of our 50 states. Those states that are more regulation oriented (i.e., states in the Northeast and on the West Coast) will provide a less hospitable environment than those that are more market oriented (states in the Southeast and the Mountain West).

The regulations imposed upon retail clinics by states vary widely. Most states require varying levels of physician supervision or collaboration with nurse practitioners. However, ten states currently permit nurse practitioners to see patients, diagnose them, and treat them without such collaboration or supervision (Christian, Dower, & O'Neil, 2007; Pearson, 2008). While one might expect those states allowing the maximum autonomy of nurse practitioners to be those states with the greatest number of nurse practitioners, such is not the case.

For example, Florida has the most retail clinics, while Minnesota also ranks high in clinic use (Tu & Cohen, 2008). However,

Minnesota ranks in the middle of states in terms of degree of nurse practitioner autonomy allowed while Florida ranks near the bottom (Lugo et al., 2007).

Several other factors are important in determining where retail clinics prosper and grow. Among the most important of these are requirements for retail clinics to be opened, requirements for owners, and requirements for licenses. The states vary widely in terms of whether they are regulated by state medical boards. Some states require regulation and other states do not (Scott, 2007). Some states license a corporation to operate clinics within the state, while other states require each clinic location to be separately licensed.

All of these state regulations impact the initial costs of starting up and long-term costs of operating retail clinics. As with any business, population density is a major factor impacting the location of clinics (Tu & Cohen, 2008). Finally, communities with a shortage of primary care physicians or lack of access to primary care services provide particularly attractive markets for retail clinics.

As retail clinics have grown, they have faced increasing scrutiny of state regulators in terms of the services they offer, who owns the clinic, and guidelines for safety and hygiene. Those states that are more heavily regulated are likely to see fewer retail clinics. Previously state regulators provided extensive hygiene and safety waivers for retail clinics. More recently they have become more restrictive. For example, in New York state there is an investigation of business relationships between drugstore companies and retail clinic providers. The purpose is to determine whether clinics attempt to send patients to pharmacies in retail settings where these clinics are located (Kershaw, 2007).

Rhode Island does not allow any retail clinics despite recent attempts by MinuteClinic (Seward, 2007). California now requires that only physicians own retail clinics, and Florida requires all retail clinic to indicate whether or not a physician will be providing the clinic services. On the other hand, some states (Texas and Wyoming) are actually beginning to loosen previous restrictions on retail clinics as well as the legal functions of nurse practitioners. Massachusetts has imposed limits on the number of patient visits to a retail clinic in a given time period due to skepticism among state regulators that such clinics provide high standards of care (Seward, 2007).

The Massachusetts Public Health Council voted to pass a set of regulations governing retail clinics in 2008 (Rhea, 2009). The new rules require retail clinics to provide an electronic record of patient visits as well as access to the patient's electronic records for each patient's primary care physician. A new medical director has been appointed to oversee clinical regulation of the clinics. Under the new regulations, retail clinics will not be granted any waivers. Obviously, Massachusetts is not a fertile state for growth of retail clinics.

Recently the Federal Trade Commission (FTC) has decided that retail clinic regulations supported by doctors in Illinois are anti-competitive and bad for consumers. The FTC letter criticizes a bill pending in the Illinois state legislature that would require permits for the facilities, limit their capacity for advertising, and mandate greater physician involvement in their operations. The letter indicated the proposed state requirements would create a competitive advantage for traditional providers by putting retail clinics at a disadvantage. Moreover, there would be no benefits for consumers that would offset this anticompetitive move. As a result, state health officials in Massachusetts dropped proposals to regulate retail clinic ads. Some believe that this decision is a setback for physician efforts to stymie the growth of retail clinics.

CONCLUSIONS

The impact of retail clinics on provider and nonprovider major stakeholders varies somewhat from state to state. Regulatory barriers vary from minimal to highly significant in different states, and as a result, many states still do not have any retail clinics while other states have hundreds.

It should also be emphasized that the impact of retail clinics on stakeholders will also vary depending upon how that stakeholder chooses to relate to and manage retail clinics. For example, if primary care physicians and specialists develop formal, collaborative relationships with retail clinics, they may actually enhance their revenues. They may choose to be adversarial and negatively impact retail clinics through federal and state political and regulatory processes. They may invest a lot of resources in such processes to the detriment of their own patients and the general public.

The long-term impact of retail clinics will be a function not only of what retailers and clinic providers do, but also the response of the various stakeholders to their initiatives. Thus far, the retailers and their clinic providers have been quite responsive to criticisms and suggestions from the medical community. Examples include electronic medical records and evidence-based medicine. As long as the stakeholders do not attempt to eliminate the competition of retail clinics through unsupported criticism regarding quality and patient safety, the future of collaborative relationships could be very bright.

REFERENCES

American Academy of Family Physicians. (2006). *America's family physicians urge retail health clinics to put patients' health first*. http://www.aafp.org/online/en/home/media/releases/2006/20060622retailhlth.html (accessed May 27, 2009).

American Academy of Family Physicians. (2007). *Desired attributes of retail health clinics*. http://www.aafp.org/online/en/home/policy/policies/r/retailhealthclinics.html (accessed July 9, 2008).

American Academy of Pediatrics. (2006). *AAP principles concerning retail-based clinics*. American Academy of Pediatrics Web site. http://www.aap.org/advocacy/releases/rbc.pdf#search=%22american%20academy%20of%20pediatrics%20principles%22 (accessed October 10, 2006).

Armstrong, D. (2008, May 7). Health clinics inside stores likely to slow their growth. *Wall Street Journal*.

AtlantiCare sees retail clinics as one more way to touch patients, and an opportunity to learn about a new way of offering care. (2007). *The Journal of Healthcare Contracting*. http://www.jhconline.com/article-janfeb2007-touchpoint.asp (accessed May 27, 2009).

Bachman, J. (2006). What do retail clinics mean for family medicine? *Family Practice Management, 13*(5), 19–20.

Bagchi, S. (2008, February 1). Mayo Clinic enters retail care business. *Health Care News*. http://www.heartland.org/policybot/results.html?articleid=22571.

Bodenheimer, T. (2008). Coordinating care—A perilous journey through the health care system. *New England Journal of Medicine, 358*(10), 1064–1071.

Bohmer, R. (2007). The rise of in-store clinics—Threat or opportunity? *New England Journal of Medicine, 356*(8), 765–768.

Bohmer, R., & Groberg, J. P. (2003). QuickMedx Inc. *Harvard Business School Case Study 9-603-049*.

Christian, S., Dower, C., & O'Neil, E. (2007). *Chart overview of nurse practitioner scopes of practice in the United States*. San Francisco: Center for the Health Professions.

Cunningham, P. J., & Felland, L. E. (2008, June). *Falling behind: Americans' access to medical care deteriorates, 2003–2007*, Tracking Report No. 19. Washington, DC: Center for Studying Health System Change.

Deloitte Center for Health Solutions. (2008). Retail clinics: Facts, trends, and implications. http://www.deloitte.com/centerforhealth solutions (accessed May 19, 2009).

Farber, J., Siu, A., & Bloom, P. (2007). How much time do physicians spend providing care outside of office visits? *Annals of Internal Medicine, 147*(10), 693–698.

Finarelli, M., & Pillai, N. (2007). *Retail health clinics*. Hospitals and Health Networks. http://www.hhnmag.com/hhnmag_app/jsp/article display.jsp?dcrpath=HHNMAG/Article/data/05MAY2007/ 070515HHN_Online_Finarelli&domain=HHNMAG (accessed May 27, 2009).

Florida Hospital Association. (2005). FHA task force on addressing the crisis in emergency care. http://www.fha.org/edreportonly.pdf (accessed December 1, 2009).

Goldstein, J. (2007). Some health systems out to beat retailers at clinic game. *Wall Street Journal Health Blog* (accessed July 14, 2008).

Hansen-Turton, T., Ryan, S., Miller, K., Counts, M., & Nash, D. B. (2007). Convenient care clinics: The future of accessible health care. *Disease Management, 10*(2), 61–73.

Japsen, B. (2007, June 25). AMA takes on retail clinics. *Chicago Tribune*.

Kershaw, S. (2007). *Drug store clinics spread, and scrutiny grows*. http:// nytimes.com/2007/08/23/nyregion/23clinic.html?_r=2&roef= slogin&pagewanted= (accessed May 27, 2009).

Lugo, N. R., O'Grady, E. T., Hodnicki, D. R., et al. (2007). Ranking state NP regulation: Practice environment and consumer healthcare choice. *American Journal for Nurse Practitioners, 11*(4), 8–24.

Malvey, D., & Fottler, M. D. (2006). The retail revolution in health care: Who will win and who will lose? *Health Care Management Review, 31*(3), 168–178.

Mattioli, D. (2009, May 26). More small firms drop health care. *Wall Street Journal*, B1, B4.

Mehrotra, A., Wang, M. C., Lave, J. R., Adams, J. L., & McGlynn, E. A. (2008). Retail clinics, primary care physicians, and emergency departments: A comparison of physician business. *Health Affairs, 27*(5), 1275–1282.

Pearson, L. J. (2008, February 12). The Pearson report. *American Journal for Nurse Practitioners* (2).

Retail-Based Clinical Policy Work Group. (2006). AAP principles concerning retail-based clinics. *Pediatrics, 118*(6), 2561–2562.

Rhea, S. (2009). Mass panel sets rules for limited care clinics. *Modern Healthcare.com: Daily Dose*.

Schmit, J. (2006). Could walk-in retail clinics help slow rising health costs? *USA Today.* http://www.usatoday.com/money/industries/health/ 2006-08-24-walk-in-clinic-usat_x.htm (accessed December 1, 2009).

Scott, M. K. (2007, September). *Health Care in the Express Lane: Retail Clinics Go Mainstream*. Report to the California Health Care Foundation.

Seward, Z. M. (2007, August 9). States boost scrutiny of drugstore clinics. *Wall Street Journal*, D1, D2.

Spencer, J. (2005, October 5). Getting your health care at Wal-Mart. *Wall Street Journal*, D1, D5.

Tu, H. T., & Cohen, G. R. (2008, December). Checking up on retail based health clinics: Is the boom ending? *The Commonwealth Fund. Issues Brief No. 1199*. New York: The Commonwealth Fund.

Zieger, A. (2008). FTC slams IL physicians' retail clinic rules. *Fierce Healthcare*. http://www.fiercehealthcare.com/story/ftc-slams-il-physicians-retail-clinic-rules/2008-06-16 (accessed May 27, 2009).

Chapter 8

The Business of Health Care

OVERVIEW

The health care crisis in the United States has also become a business crisis. When CEOs are surveyed, they identify health benefits costs as the number one economic pressure (Berry, Mirabito, & Berwick, 2004, p. 56). Two United States senators, Ron Wyden (D) from Oregon and Bob Bennett (R) from Utah, sponsored legislation in the 110th Congress (the Healthy Americans Act), which in part would modernize employer-sponsored health insurance to permit employers and employees to participate in reducing health care costs. The senators observed the following in the journal *Health Affairs*:

> America currently spends enough on health care to pay for health coverage for all Americans. For the amount we spend collectively today, we could hire a physician for every seven families in America. (Wyden & Bennett, 2008, p. 692)

The senators' calculations assumed $2.2 trillion in health care spending and a family size of four.

This observation has a lot of shock value, especially for Americans who have little or no access to health care. But it is also upsetting for employers to be captive in a system that depends on employer-sponsored insurance. Employer-sponsored insurance was an innovation of the 1940s. At that time, there were wage and price controls that prohibited employers from offering higher salaries. In order to attract workers, employers began to offer health benefits instead of wages. The federal tax code supported this design by permitting employers to exempt the cost of health insurance with pretax dollars. Over time, health benefits have become a standard offering for most employers.

However, the cost of health benefits has been growing to the point where it has created a conundrum for employers. If they do not offer coverage, they may not be able to attract a talented workforce. Yet the high costs present a competitive disadvantage to employers. The rising costs affect productivity and the ability of employers to compete and survive in the global marketplace. It also undermines the ability of small businesses to offer comprehensive coverage and for working families to afford it. In response to escalating costs, many employers have eliminated or reduced health care benefits for employees. Others have eliminated jobs or relocated operations outside the United States (Wyden & Bennett, 2008).

Employers recognize that there is a link between the health of their employees and profits. Studies by the National Business Group on Health and Watson Wyatt Worldwide, "2007/2008 Staying@Work," showed that effective health and productivity management programs yielded more revenue per employee (20 percent) and greater shareholder returns (57 percent) (Wojcik, 2007). Thus it is incumbent on employers to find ways to keep their employers healthy at a reduced cost to the organization.

As this chapter illustrates, the business sector is not sitting back, waiting for the government to *fix* the health care system. Employers are trying different care models and innovations in an attempt to gain control over skyrocketing health care costs. And technology combined with strategic entrepreneurship appears to be creating opportunities for disrupting conventional methods for delivering primary care health services, all of which portend savings. From virtual clinic visits to telephone consultations to affordable electronic health records, the health care landscape is under construction.

EMPLOYER-BASED HEALTH CARE

Employee health benefit costs are growing faster than inflation, and they are draining profits from companies. In the United States employer-provided health insurance is the dominant form of health care coverage for workers and their families. In 2005, employers contributed approximately $420 billion, more than one-fifth of total U.S. health care expenditures in that year, for insurance premiums for employees and their dependents. In 2006, the national average of annual health cost per employee was reported to be $6,900 (Collins & Kriss, 2008, Wells, 2006). In 2007, the average annual cost for family coverage in an employer-based health plan was $12,106. This amount exceeded the average yearly earnings of a full-time worker earning minimum wage (Claxton et al., 2007).

If employers are to survive rising health care costs and remain competitive in the United States and in global markets, they must look for ways to reduce the cost of care for their employees. Employers essentially face five options: (1) give control of employee health benefits over to a national health plan, (2) continue to offer health benefits, but pass along the increasing costs to employees, (3) stop offering health benefits and let employees purchase their own coverage in private markets, (4) adopt the use of disruptive innovations such as retail health clinics and services, which have the potential to provide quality care at lower costs, and (5) use on-site clinics to offer cost effective health services.

However, some of these options face challenges. For example, a Commonwealth Fund Survey (Collins & Kriss, 2008) reported that the *public* wants employers to retain responsibility for providing health insurance or at least to continue contributing financially to securing coverage for their employees and families. Meanwhile, a recent National Business Group on Health study revealed that employees value their employer-sponsored health plans and are unwilling to purchase insurance on their own, even if given the funds to do so (Pierce, 2007). The question is what should any level of government do in terms of public policy to encourage employers in these change efforts? Thus far, the government has not provided any incentives to business, thereby leaving employers to follow their own paths.

THE ON-SITE CLINIC

Employers are meeting the challenges of rising health care costs through the adoption of a variety of innovations, including on-site clinics and retail-based health clinics. On-site medical care evokes the model of "company doctor" that was prevalent in the late nineteenth and early twentieth centuries. However, those clinics fell out of favor because the doctors were primarily serving the interests of employers (Welch, 2008). In 2009, on-site clinics represent an attempt by employers to take the lead in efforts to control health care costs and maintain a healthy workforce.

Evolution of the On-site Clinic

In the 1800s, large companies such as those that built railroads or mined coal hired company doctors to take care of their workers. They did so because the work locations were remote and doctors were otherwise unavailable. In the 1960s and 1970s, on-site clinics furnished a variety of services from wellness care to drug screenings. However, evidence about their cost effectiveness was scarce and questionable.

The reemergence of the on-site clinic in the twenty-first century reflects another disruption of primary care service delivery (Merchant Medicine, 2009a). Employers are adopting these clinics to reduce health care costs by taking care of workers before they need to receive more expensive specialty care. About 100 or more of the largest employers offer on-site primary care or preventive health services to their employees (Freudenheim, 2007).

Today's on-site clinics bear little resemblance to the original model, and they are distinct from traditional occupational health clinics that manufacturing businesses and factories have offered for on-the-job injuries and worker's compensation cases. The new on-site clinics offer basic primary care services and immunizations such as allergy and flu shots (Freudenheim, 2007). In addition, both employers and purveyors of on-site clinics congregate for workshops and annual meetings to strategize and share information at the *On-Site Employee Health Clinic Summit*, 2008 and 2009 (World Research Group, 2008).

Businesses are adopting on-site clinics because they enable them to better manage and control health care expenditures. In addition, they reduce time spent on doctors' visits by employees and in some cases promote healthier life-styles that benefit the company in the long term (Wells, 2006). However, as with retail clinics, on-site clinics in 2009 occupy a *niche* status (Kennedy, 2008). If they continue to reduce health care costs and if there is no significant health care reform, on-site clinics may end up in the *mainstream* of health care.

Models for On-Site Clinics

The type of model that an employer chooses for its on-site clinic varies widely. At one end of the spectrum, there are employers who adopt these clinics purely in anticipation of reducing health care costs. At the other end of the spectrum are companies that are more focused on developing a healthy workplace and health-conscious workers. Most employers are probably somewhere in between with a shared belief that healthy employees also affect the bottom line of their company.

In addition, some employers want employees to use the on-site clinics as their *medical home* for primary care services. Medical home is a model of coordinated primary care that occurs in one setting, usually a family practice (Barry, 2009, p. 13). These employers outwardly encourage their employees to replace their primary care physicians with clinic staff. Meanwhile, other employers are simply utilizing clinics to make sure that their employees have access to quick and affordable care. These employers look to increase productivity by reducing the time that employees spend away from their jobs for medical care visits and also to ensure that employees do not delay care because of the cost of care.

Many employers do not intend for the on-site clinic to be the medical home for their employees. For example, Intel Corporation offers basic primary care services and some preventive care at its Arizona corporate campus. Intel contracted with Take Care Health System, which is owned by Walgreens, to operate the clinics (Colliver, 2008).

But some clinics are gravitating toward creating clinics that function as the primary health care provider for their workers. One such example is Cisco Systems. Cisco Systems operates an on-site clinic at the networking equipment maker's San Jose, California, headquarters. The clinic is staffed by four family practice physicians and an internist. It also offers physical therapy, acupuncture, chiropractic services, and a pharmacy run by Walgreens. The clinic boasts amenities such as "care suites," private rooms in which patients can meet with their doctors, and choices of robes or gowns for the examination room. The clinic is part of the company's new $48 million LifeConnections Center that also includes child care and a 48,000-square-foot gym (Colliver, 2008).

Some large employers such as Quad/Graphics, the largest commercial printer in America, are also offering employees access to specialists. Quad/Graphics, which owns its on-site clinics, is also offering clinic services to other employers in the area. Meanwhile, many employers, both large and small, are essentially outsourcing clinic operations to companies such as Walgreens's Take Care Health. For example, Toyota hired Take Care Health to run its on-site clinic in San Antonio (Merchant Medicine, 2009a).

Does Size Matter?

Even though early on-site clinic ventures have focused on large employers, they can be configured to work for small employers, too (Klepper, 2008). But the evidence suggests that scale is necessary for success. Some clinic operators suggest there should be 1,000 employees in a single location, with the majority of workers signed up to use the clinic. Furthermore, there is a two to three year return (Welch, 2008; Colliver, 2008).

Industry experts and consultants Merchant Medicine (April 2009) reported that typical on-site clinics, especially those operated by the major clinic operators, have a population of 1,000 to 3,000 people at the site. The clinics are usually open full time, five days a week. They are staffed by a combination of providers, ranging from physicians to nurse practitioners and medical assistants. The clinics also usually offer extended hours one or more days a week to cover shift workers. Clinic operators typically charge a percentage management fee based on the cost of the practitioners. They also charge for physician oversight, professional liability, and some allocated costs. Reports are generated for every visit to the clinics and are usually integrated into the employer's health informatics.

What about Cost Savings?

iTrax, one of the largest proprietors and operators of on-site clinics, estimates that they produce savings in the range of 5 percent to 20 percent (Wells, 2006). SAIF Corporation, which is a worker's compensation insurance company located in Oregon, has over 800 employees at both its main facility and branch offices throughout the state. The company is in its fifteenth year of using an on-site clinic. According to Merchant Medicine (April 2, 2009), SAIF reported overall savings from 1999 to 2005 of $2.15 million.

The Pepsi Bottling Group operates 11 employee health clinics at its facilities in the United States and plans to add approximately 15 more. During 2004 and the first half of 2005, the company saved nearly $100,000 at its Baltimore clinic by having employees visit the on-site clinic instead of a doctor's office. The company also saved more than $50,000 during the same time period in replacement labor expenses for employee time off to visit the clinic (Wells, 2006).

The city of Port St. Lucie, Florida, contracted with WeCare to offer its employees primary care services. The city reported that during its first six months of operation, the clinic produced a 3.1:1

hard return on investment, with savings in primary care visits, drugs, laboratory, sick hours, and out-of-pocket employee savings (Klepper, 2008). Lowe's Companies, Inc., the home improvement retailer, also has opened on-site clinics at two distribution centers and expects to continue opening more clinics (Wells, 2006).

Outsourcing Clinic Management

Employers can hire an outside firm to set up and manage the clinic. Employees are offered incentives to use the on-site clinic, such as reduced co-payments. Some employers prefer direct contracting with providers, and there are firms that help companies negotiate and manage direct contracts with doctors and hospitals (Wells, 2006). There is also a trend toward consolidation among management companies.

National operators of retail pharmacies and retail clinics such as Walgreens and its Take Care Health Division are interested in on-site clinics in a very big way. MinuteClinic is also operating on-site clinics, but not to the extent of Take Care Health, which has been aggressive. In 2008, Walgreens, an active participant in retail clinics, took another turn in the primary care delivery system by acquiring two of the largest and well-established firms that provide on-site clinics, iTrax and Whole Health Management (Klepper, 2008). CHD Meridian is a wholly owned subsidiary of iTrax and provides workplace health care services to more than 100 companies nationwide. Its client base ranges from large financial institutions to manufacturers of consumer products and auto parts (Garcia, Powers, & Clarke, 2008). Whole Health management is regarded as a leading operator of on-site clinics and wellness and fitness centers for large self-insured corporations in the United States since 1981. Its client base is diverse ranging from Scotts Miracle-Gro, the largest marketer of consumer lawn and garden products, to Freddie Mac, one of the nation's largest investors in residential mortgages (Crate & Siefkin, 2005).

In addition, Walgreens located the two companies in a new Health and Wellness Division along with its retail clinic operator, Take Care Health. Walgreens also launched a major employer-focused initiative called "Complete Care and Well-Being. With this purchase, 370 on-site clinics were added along with 180 new clients, some of which are among the largest employers in the United States, i.e., Toyota, Sprint/Nextel, Lowe's, Pitney Bowes, Florida

Power & Light, Freddie Mac, Qualcomm, and Fidelity (Wohl & Zimmerman, 2009; Merchant Medicine, 2009a).

From large private companies such as Disney and Toyota to local county governments, clinic management companies are engaged in serving a variety of clients. What follows are some examples of the diversity of clients that are served.

Disney

Walt Disney Parks and Resorts opened its on-site clinic, a $6 million facility in 2008 to serve more than 40,000 employees and their dependents (Welch, 2008). The facility is intended to offer its employees one-stop shopping for primary care (Balancia, 2007). The 15,000-square-foot facility is operated by Walgreens's Take Care Health Systems. It offers primary care, urgent care, preventive care, a pharmacy, a medical laboratory, and radiology (Powers, 2008).

Toyota

Toyota's U.S. health care costs doubled to more than $11,000 annually per worker during the period 2001–2006. Consequently, Toyota is looking to reduce health care costs by using the concept of the on-site clinic (Healthcare News, 2006). Toyota constructed its on-site medical center called the Toyota Family Medical Center at its truck factory in San Antonio. The cost of the 20,000-square-foot facility was $9 million, which is a substantial investment. The medical center is operated and managed by Take Care Health Systems, which is a division of Walgreens.

The medical center provides employees with basic care services. It has helped Toyota reduce big-ticket medical expenses, including referrals to highly paid specialists, emergency room visits, and the use of costly brand name drugs. Toyota has also realized productivity gains because workers do not leave the plant to visit a doctor. About 60 percent of the San Antonio staff use the on-site facility (Welch, 2008).

Public Sector Clients (Local Government)

Local county governments have adopted employee medical clinics. For example, in Rutherford County, Tennessee, a trailer located at a school site functions as a clinic. It is staffed by a doctor and medical clinic personnel. It offers primary care services to school district employees who are on an insurance plan. Employees can make an appointment by telephone or electronically. One teacher spent 30 minutes at the clinic, instead of missing a day of school, and returned with a 30-day supply of an antibiotic for a sinus infection. The clinic is owned and operated by a Brentwood, Tennessee–based company, CareHere service. The school district has two additional clinics in the county and anticipates savings of $1 million in the first year of clinic service. In addition to saving money on prescription drugs, they expect to reduce the cost for substitute teachers (Broden, 2004).

In addition to the school district employees, the clinics also service county employees, retirees, and their spouses who are on the county's health insurance plan. County employees do not pay anything when they visit the clinic. And the clinics also offer preventative services. Sumner County, Tennessee, operates a similar program with the same company, CareHere, to run its clinics. The county reported healthier employees with higher attendance records that saved the county money (Booth, 2005).

CareHere operates employer-based clinics in both private and public sectors in more than six states. It runs employer-based clinics for city employees in Ocoee and Palm Bay, Florida. Ocoee city workers and their dependents have access to free doctor visits, free prescription drugs, and a clinic across the street from City Hall. City employees, about 340, are able to see a primary care physician during their work hours. The clinic has three exam rooms, a digital x-ray room, and a drug dispensary. In Palm Bay, Florida, city employees have access to a similar type of clinic that is located in a shopping mall about a mile from City Hall. However, Palm Bay employees must visit the clinic on their own time (Wessel, 2008).

In Fairfield, Alabama, the doctor's office is also at City Hall and the clinic is also run by CareHere. The city government faced $170,000 annual increase in health care costs and opted for a on-site clinic to keep employees healthier and reduce health care costs. City employees report that they enjoy the convenience and also visiting with the doctor for an average of 16 minutes. The national average is between six and eight minutes (Plott, 2007).

Employer-Owned Clinics

Some employers have experimented with owning their own clinics. One example of a long-term clinic operation and a success story is the Rosen Clinic in Orlando, Florida. In the early 1990s, when Hillary Clinton was creating her national health plan, Harris Rosen, the owner and president of Rosen Hotel and Resorts in Orlando, Florida, self-insured his company and put together a health plan that centered around a company doctor and clinic. The plan offered employees free doctor visits with no deductibles or co-payments, annual physicals and preventive care, prenatal and well-baby care, along with pharmacy and dental benefits. Rosen calculated that his plan cut his per-employee health cost from $2,223 to $850, whereas Clinton's plan would have added at least $300 to employee costs and would have lessened the quality of care for his workers (Howard, 2007).

Between 1996 and 2004, Florida's population increased by 3 million, but 130,000 businesses in Florida dropped health coverage. Meanwhile, the Rosen health clinic continued to save the company money and provide quality health care to employees and their families. The company's clinic reports two full time physicians on staff, two nurse practitioners, and a support staff. There is an on-site laboratory and x-ray facilities (Howard, 2007). Employees are permitted to visit the company clinic while still "on the clock," meaning that they will not lose time for attending to their health needs. The plan also includes specialists and health facilities within the UnitedHealthcare network (Howard, 2007). In an industry in which even high end hotels experience turnover rates between 50 percent and 60 percent, Rosen's employee turnover rate is about 15 percent (Berry, Mirabito, & Berwick, 2004).

The Future of On-site Clinics

On-site clinics were also attempted in the 1950s and peaked in the 1970s, when they gradually began to be eliminated. They were eliminated because employers either did not find them cost effective or found them ineffective for other reasons such as redundancy. For example, Ford Motor Company discontinued its on-site clinics because it felt that most employees preferred to go to their own doctors for primary care (Freudenheim, 2007). However, today patients have less of a relationship with their physicians than in the past, mostly because of managed care. Under managed care, physicians were transformed into *providers* and patients into *customers* and insurers occupied the spot of middleman (Mahar, 2006; Brownlee, 2007).

The new model of employer-sponsored on-site clinics differs from past endeavors in that it attempts to link employee health and performance, usually by creating a self-insured health care system for its employees. The goal of cost reduction is combined with a focus on employee health that provides for enhanced employee performance and productivity (Wells, 2006).

A 2007 study by Watson Wyatt Worldwide, a human resource consulting firm, reported that 33 percent of 275 organizations that collectively employ more than 4.9 million workers have implemented on-site medical clinics or plan to do so within the year (Wojcik, 2007). From Toyota, Nextel, Sprint, Pepsi Bottling Group, Credit Suisse, to most recently Disney, the list of private sector businesses that have opened or expanded on-site clinics is growing (Balancia, 2008; Freudenheim, 2007). Furthermore, it is not just private sector employers that are jumping on the on-site clinic bandwagon. Local governments are also adopting these clinics as a means of reducing their insurance costs and improving workers' health (Wessel, 2008).

In addition, insurers such as Cigna and Aetna have also recognized that the proliferation of on-site clinics poses a potential threat. Because insurers often operate on-site disease management clinics, they could face competition directly from employer-based clinics that refer patients to these programs instead of those offered by the patient's health insurer. Thus, insurers are faced with decisions to partner with the employer and clinic provider in order to avoid competition (Freudenheim, 2007).

Employer benefits for adopting on-site clinics are both tangible and intangible, including cost savings and improving quality of care by such actions as minimizing time spent on doctor's visits, decreasing or eliminating visits to more costly facilities, expediting recovery, reducing absenteeism, assisting in the management of chronic conditions, and encouraging the maintenance of better health. In addition, on-site clinics hold the promise of increasing risk management efforts especially with regard to on-the-job treatment of workplace injuries and helping employers to attract and retain highly skilled and productive workers. Employee benefits from on-site clinics include enhanced access and quality plus reduced out-of-pocket expense.

HEALTH INFORMATION TECHNOLOGY

Dr. Robert Solow, an MIT economics professor and also a Nobel Prize winner, suggested that Walmart was mostly responsible for

U.S. productivity gains from 1995 to 2000. Walmart invested heavily in information systems that contributed to its ability to out-perform competitors and force them to play catch up. But it was not just the technology; it was how Walmart used information systems to support innovation, leverage productivity, and increase customer satisfaction (Beckham, 2002, p. 38). Thus when Walmart and other retailers moved into health care markets, they did so with a view toward using information technology to support retail clinics and other innovative efforts.

The key to retailers' disruptive innovations is their use of technology. Retail clinics use electronic health records and standardized digital protocols. Newer clinic models include telemedicine components. Meanwhile, other entrepreneurs are reinventing a variety of services online, from laboratory work to physician consultations.

Dossia

In 2006, five of the largest employers in the United States announced plans to give employees their very own electronic medical record for life. The record will be their property, and they can take them when they travel, change jobs, or visit doctors. The five large employers behind this endeavor are Walmart, BP America, Intel Corporation, Pitney Bowes, and Applied Materials. These companies believe that rising health care costs pose a threat to America's competitiveness and therefore are committed to playing a role in helping the health care system to improve efficiency and effectiveness. They have established a nonprofit consortium whose goal is to develop "Dossia" a Web-based framework through which 2.5 million U.S. employees, their dependents, and also retirees can maintain lifelong personal health records (Dossia, 2006).

Dossia is a multimillion dollar initiative that is being underwritten by these large employers. The effort shows that business is taking the lead by putting its own money on the line (Hoover, 2006). By giving their employees their own records, health care paperwork and administrative costs should be reduced. Furthermore, medical errors and duplicative care may also be reduced. Omnimedix Institute of Portland, Oregon, an independent nonprofit organization, will maintain the health records and gather information from insurers, pharmacies, doctors, and other providers (Freking, 2006; Dossia, 2006).

Meanwhile, the American Medical Association (AMA) is working with Compuware Corporation to develop a Web-based service that offers doctors electronic prescribing as well as up to-date reference material and other resources. The service is aimed at making it easier for physicians to adopt electronic health record technology (Associated Press, 2009).

Electronic Health Records

The health care industry as a whole has been slow to adopt electronic health records technology even though it promises to make the health care system more efficient and eliminate waste (*Economist*, 2006). Most health care organizations have tended to use information technology for financial systems, including the production of financial reports, none of which contributes to increased productivity or customer service (Beckham, 2009). A survey by the American Hospital Association (AHA) found that relatively few hospitals, between 2 percent and 12 percent use electronic health records (zz_Ferris, November 12, 2008).

Years from now it will probably be shown that retailers such as Walmart raised the bar for health care and compelled hospitals and health systems as well as physicians to play catch up when it came to information technology. For example, in March 2009, Walmart announced plans to market a digital health records system that will enable physicians to adopt an affordable electronic health record for their offices. Even though the use of electronic health records is widespread among large group physician practices, most physician practices are small and few use computerized records (Lohr, 2009).

Past estimates showed that about 24 percent of doctors used electronic health records. However, this took into account billing and computerized systems that were unrelated to health care (zz_Ferris, June 18, 2008). Physicians in small practices have been challenged in adopting electronic health records by the lack of affordability and also technical support. Also, vendors have tended to avoid smaller practices because of the cost in selling to them. Consulting group Avalere Health reported that it could cost about $124,000 for a single doctor to upgrade to the electronic health record in the next five years (Lohr, 2009; Perrone, 2009).

Walmart partnered with Dell for computers and eClinicalWorks, a private company, for software. Walmart will offer physicians a package deal through its Sam's Club division that essentially bundles hardware, software, installation, maintenance, and training. Walmart is expected to be able to undercut rival health information technology suppliers and offer digital systems for about $44,000. In addition, the financial incentives in the current administration plan, with more than $40,000 allocated per physician to install and use health records, could accelerate sales (Lohr, 2009; Perrone, 2009).

Digital Doctor Visits

Technology has taken medicine out of the doctor's office. Retailers such as Walmart have been quick to explore the idea of a digital doctor's visit using their in-store clinics. Walmart is already testing a telemedicine version of the retail clinic at six of its Houston area stores. The first "Walk-In Telemedicine Health Care" clinics are operated by My Healthy Access, Inc., a retail clinic company operator, and NuPhysicia LLC, a commercial entity that was created in 2007 to utilize telemedicine methods developed by the University of Texas Medical Branch at Galveston. Unlike retail clinics, the telemedicine health care clinics will be staffed by paramedics and physicians linked to the clinics via video technology (Perin, 2008).

More companies are beginning to offer telemedicine consultations. These services are the next step in the delivery of health care through the telephone, Web, or other telecommunications technologies (Lawton, 2009). These types of consultations are appealing to many people, especially uninsured patients as well as others who have been affected by the recession. The cost of a consult is far less than an in-person visit to the doctor (Lawton, 2009). For example, America Well offers an online service to patients in Hawaii's Blue Cross Blue Shield. The cost is $10 for a ten minute consultation (Lawton, 2009). Physicians can view patient personal health records using Microsoft's HealthVault and even prescribe medication over the Web.

There are a variety of services that permit physicians to communicate directly and remotely with a patient. In addition to America Well, there is SwiftMD, which is available in New York and New Jersey, and Dallas-based TelaDoc that is available nationwide. LivePerson offers Web chat and telephone access to a wide variety of health professionals including physicians for a flat fee (Zieger, 2009). However, physician-licensing regulations and health plans vary across states, and the availability of electronic consultations is restricted as a result (Lawton, 2009).

Blue Cross Blue Shield of Minnesota is testing a virtual clinic model, using American Well's service, Online Care, with its 10,000 employees and family members. There will be live interactions with physicians and other medical care providers. The virtual clinics at the on-site clinic will emphasize treatment for common illnesses, monitor care for patients with chronic illnesses, and offer preventive and wellness care. The insurer hopes to make online care available to employer groups by 2010 (Merrill, 2009).

Creating Online Health Care Communities

In 2008, the University of California–Merced announced the opening of six telemedicine centers in rural and underserved communities in the state's San Joaquin Valley. These sites have some of the worst ratios of doctor to patients in the state, with one licensed physician per 686 residents. This is compared with one physician for 379 residents elsewhere. The university offers consultations with specialists in addition to primary care services. Video technology is used to link out-of-area doctors with local patients. The project was funded by about $1 million in grants, including $500,000 from AT&T (Goldeen, 2008).

Richard Scott of Solantic and Allison Guimard of Alijor.com have cofounded an online health care community that connects patients and health care providers. Alijor allows physicians and hospitals to post prices, hours, services, insurance plans, and other information for free and similarly permits patients to search the providers for free. More than 60,000 physicians and hospitals post prices on Alijor (Wikipedia, 2008).

Physicians have gained compensation from insurers for online consultations with patients, which may support their interest in them. The consultations are for simple health questions that might be answered over the phone, but for which the physician usually does not get reimbursed. Aetna completed a three-state test pilot program that reimbursed physician consultations and eventually took the program nationwide. Cigna also has plans to compensate doctors for Web visits. Both Aetna and Cigna contract with a company called RelayHealth that has built a secure online system for physician-patient consults. Patients typically pay the same co-pay for an online consult as they do for an office visit. Insurers pay doctors less for a Web consult, about $25–$35 (Goldstein, 2008).

ENTREPRENEURS

There are a number of entrepreneurs who have established businesses aimed at reducing the cost of health care. Below are some highlights of prominent entrepreneurs and a description of some of the retail businesses that have emerged.

RediClinic

Steve Case, who founded America Online Inc. (AOL), has gotten into health care in a big way. He launched Revolution Health Group, which houses a number of start-up health companies. Case's goal is to build the leading comprehensive consumer-driven health company that puts patients at the center of the health care system. Patients will face more choices, more convenience, and more control over their health care.

RediClinic is an example of one of the vehicles that is driving Case's health care revolution. RediClinic, formerly known as Inter-Fit, operates clinics in Walmart stores and drugstores such as Duane Reade in New York. RediClinic also partners with hospitals and health systems and offers services tailored to employers (Yang, 2005; Clark, 2005; Revolution Health Group, 2005). In its year-end review for 2008, Merchant Marine reported RediClinic with 21 clinics. This made it the largest privately backed proprietor of retail clinics (Merchant Medicine, 2009b). RediClinic also has a contract to see TRICARE beneficiaries at its facilities located inside Walmart stores in the greater Richmond, Virginia, market. TRICARE's provider network offers health care services to active duty and retired military personnel and their families (Business Wire, 2008).

Solantic

Solantic is a privately held company that was established in 2001 as a provider of physician-staffed, convenient walk-in and urgent health care. Solantic operates clinics in Florida: freestanding urgent care clinics as well as retail clinics in Walmart. Solantic obtained a $100 million investment from a private equity firm, Welsh, Carson, Anderson & Stowe in 2007. The funds will be used to open at least 40 more clinics and to establish a national health care brand as the leading provider of urgent care and other health care services (Strupp, 2007).

Richard Scott, who founded Solantic, eventually intends to take the company public within the next five years. Scott is an attorney and also the founder, former chairman, and CEO of Columbia/ HCA Healthcare Corporation, one of the largest for-profit hospital companies in America (Strupp, 2007). Prior to his involvement with Columbia/HCA, Scott had represented hospitals and hospital chains as a lawyer. He had no experience in hospital management and had never operated a hospital or other medical facility (Wikipedia, 2008).

Thus far, Solantic has differentiated itself from other retail clinics by staffing with physicians. In 2008, Solantic tested the use of health debit cards that were purchased for $299, but offered $400 worth of care (Immediate Care Business, 2009). In addition, Solantic has offered a flu shot guarantee that promises to refund the price of a flu shot if the patient comes down with the flu (Solantic, 2008a).

Hospitals and Health Systems

Are hospital systems the new entrepreneurial class? In the 1970s and 1980s, hospitals and health systems invested in non–health care ventures that were beyond their scope of expertise. For example, they purchased Dude Ranches in Montana and other non–health care related enterprises, most of which failed. Hospitals must have learned their lesson because now they are sticking to health care enterprises.

Hospital systems are partnering with retail giants such as Walmart and privately backed companies such as RediClinic in retail clinic ventures. Instead of competing with retail clinics, hospitals are collaborating with them. They are using the retail clinic as an *entry point* to their network of services as well as their physician base. In doing so, they have the opportunity to increase their market share and revenues. Retail clinics backed by hospital systems were identified as the fastest-growing segment of the 2008 retail health care market (Harris, 2008).

Nationwide, about one in ten retail clinics has a hospital connection (Freudenheim, 2009). For example, Walmart reports more than 25 hospital connected clinics in their stores. The prestigious Cleveland Clinic is collaborating with CVS drugstores in Northeastern Ohio. Academic health centers also are part of the trend toward linkages with retail clinics. Wisconsin-based Aurora Health Care, which represents an integrated academic health system, operates 19 clinics, more than any other health system. Similarly, Baylor Health Care System in Dallas has also partnered with a retail clinic company, MedBasics. And Geisinger Health Care in Pennsylvania operates five retail clinics in that state (Harris, 2008).

Unlike the majority of hospitals, the Mayo Clinic opened its own stand-alone storefront clinic called Mayo Express Care in a strip mall. The clinic is staffed by nurse practitioners who work closely with Mayo Health System physicians. Furthermore, the clinic is directly connected to the Mayo electronic health record so the clinic's files are accessible from a variety of entry points: primary care, urgent care, and emergency care (Robeznieks, 2007).

Thus far, hospitals and health systems have mostly collaborated with retailers to offer retail clinics. They also have an opportunity to capture part of the employer market, but they face challenges in doing so. The hospital must be able to offer remote clinic management, provide primary care staffing of the on-site clinic, and offer ancillary service support as required. In addition, the hospital must utilize electronic medical records, which may be a major challenge because so few hospitals have adopted electronic health records. Finally, the hospital must be able to recruit physicians to participate in these ventures (LaPenna, 2009). This will not be easy as physicians mostly have resisted collaborating with retail clinic ventures.

OTHER RETAIL BUSINESS VENTURES

What follows are some examples of other retail business ventures that are designed to offer convenient and affordable care.

Walk-in Doctor's Offices

The American Medical Association reported that a number of physicians are expanding their office hours or forming their own clinics to compete with retailers. The competition has led to the development of new retail spin-offs of expanded physician services. One such spin-off, Consumer Health Services, Inc., was founded by a former investor of MinuteClinic. It offers doctor's offices at selected drugstores in the New York City area (Associated Press, 2007a).

On-Demand Laboratory Tests

A number of laboratory services are available without a doctor's visit. HS Labs (BloodWorksUSA.com) permits patients to register online, pay a fee, and then drop by one of their nationwide collection points. At the collection point, a technician draws a blood sample. The costs are much less expensive than those furnished in a doctor's office or private laboratory. DirectLabs.com offers a similar battery of tests. Results are available online or by mail within a few days (Herrick, 2006).

Cash-Friendly Practices

Physicians who are looking for alternatives to the high overhead costs and low reimbursements associated with third-party payment can use CashDoctor.com. It is a loosely structured national network of a variety of health care providers, including physicians, dentists, pharmacies, hospitals, and outpatient facilities that accept cash payments. The providers offer lower prices because they avoid the expense of insurance billing (Herrick, 2006).

Personal Health Advising Firms

When Senator Ted Kennedy was diagnosed with a brain tumor, he received the advice of his doctors at the prestigious Massachusetts General Hospital. The doctors identified the tumor as inoperable. The senator then reached out to a physician friend who investigated experimental treatments and spoke with leading cancer specialists. In the end, Senator Kennedy left Boston and had an experimental surgical procedure performed at Duke University Hospital. He then returned to Boston for follow-up treatments.

Opportunities to access the best medical advice are not limited to famous people. However, they are limited to the more affluent. Since 2002, personal health advising firms have opened. Their customers include people who pay fees ranging from $150 an hour to $100,000 a year to obtain advice on the best doctors and treatments for their illnesses. Private health consultants are aimed at filling the gap in health care between overworked primary care doctors who have less and less time to spend with patients and patients who want more information and coordination of care. PinnacleCare, a Baltimore health advising firm, is an example of this type of firm. It seeks the wealthy as clients. Its fees range from $7,000 to $100,000 a year, not including an initial sign-up fee. It offers a standard family membership of $10,000 (Wertheimer, 2008).

Concierge or Boutique Care

Some physicians offer more personalized care for an annual fee. The fee ensures that the patient will have quick access to physicians and be able to spend more time with them.

Retail Health Insurance

Blue Cross Blue Shield of Florida opened its first "insurance store" in Jacksonville, Florida, in 2007. In doing so, it began a test of the retail selling of insurance. Within a year, the insurer opened a second store in south Florida, located in a shopping center in Pembroke Pines. This retail approach reflects the insurer's belief that consumers should be able to purchase their health insurance much the same way they buy a cellular phone. It also highlights the increasingly competitive environment among insurance companies.

Prescription Drug Business

While MinuteClinic, Take Care, and other operators are targeting on-site clinics, Walmart's approach for employers appears to be through lowering the cost of prescription drugs. Walmart conducted a pilot test program with Caterpillar that has yielded promising results and is in talks with other employers.

Caterpillar contracted to buy prescription drugs for its employees directly through Walmart. This process is different from the way most employers purchase drugs, which is through a middleman known as a pharmacy benefits manager. By eliminating the middleman, Walmart has been able to significantly lower prescription drug costs for Caterpillar (Jones, 2009).

Walmart has had dramatic success in lowering drug costs for consumers. In 2006, Walmart introduced the $4 generic drug program, which eventually was matched by other pharmacy retailers such as Walgreens and discount retailers, including Target and Costco (Maurer, 2006). Eventually, Walmart hopes to drive down drug costs for the entire health industry (Jones, 2009).

Airport Clinics

Airport clinics represent a new access portal to primary care services and a potential growth market for retail health services. Most take insurance, including Medicare. Clinics operated by Solantic offer some urgent care services in addition to basic care (Yu, 2008). Many offer immunizations and flu shots to passengers once they have cleared security. In 2007, airport clinics in Atlanta, Chicago, Denver, Newark, and San Francisco sold about 15,000 flu shots that cost between $15 to $35, depending on the airport (Associated Press, 2007a).

Retail Clinics and Urgent Care Centers

The National Business Group on Health (NGBH) has come out in support of employer use of retail clinics because they offer employees quick, convenient, and affordable preventative and primary care services. They also offer vaccinations and diagnostic screenings for chronic conditions such as high blood pressure and diabetes. The group's board of directors, including five physician members, reviewed research reports and publications about retail clinics before recommending that the clinics were worth supporting (Hunt, 2007).

Even though much of the attention concerning convenient care has focused on retail clinics, urgent care clinics have been experiencing dramatic growth. Observers are noting that urgent care centers actually complement rather than compete with retail clinics (FierceHealthcare, 2007b). Retail clinics are for basic health problems such as earaches and immunizations. Urgent care clinics are for acute problems that go beyond the scope of the retail clinic. These would include sprains, minor burns, cuts requiring stitches, and suspected broken bones (Consumer Reports, 2009).

Some hospitals and health systems are moving into urgent care and operating their own centers in order to reduce overcrowding in their emergency departments. For example, Duke University Medical Center observed that people did not have access to care outside normal business hours and were using the emergency department as a default provider. It set up two urgent care clinics that helped stabilize emergency department admissions at about 58,000 patients per year since the clinics opened (Traugot, 2007).

Emergency Departments

Overcrowded emergency departments have been searching for ways to reduce the numbers of nonurgent care patients that they see. Retail clinics and urgent care clinics appear to offer these departments an opportunity to proactively divert patients to other care providers before they arrive at the emergency room. A study by the Center for Studying Health System Change ("Safety Net Hospital Emergency Departments: Creating Safety Values for Non-Urgent Care") reported on hospital efforts to screen patients in advance and refer them to facilities that offered primary care services (Felland et al., 2008).

RISE OF CORPORATE ENTERPRISE IN HEALTH SERVICES

In the twentieth century, doctors managed to maintain their autonomy and tradition of independent professionalism. While large corporations were expanding and dominating economic life, doctors managed to escape corporate and bureaucratic control in their own practices. There has been a dramatic increase, however, in a movement by physicians toward the corporate organization of doctors. For example, doctors own companies that contract a variety of staff and services to hospitals, emergency departments, clinics, and health plans. More recently, doctors have been participating in businesses that offer telephone and Web consultations.

In the past, doctors have fought against corporate control. Their relationship with the patient has made this possible, and consequently doctors have worked hard to sustain a relationship where no one gets between the physician and the patient, including powerful insurance companies. During the 1990s, managed care organizations such as HMOs attempted to insinuate themselves in the physician-patient relationship. HMOs restricted patients from seeking specialty care and often overruled physician treatment plans, including prescriptions for diagnostic tests and drugs. The end result was a backlash by patients.

The backlash was so widespread that managed care organizations eventually loosened controls. Today, doctors use hospital facilities, equipment, and personnel to treat and care for their patients, yet continue to do so at no charge. In addition, they remain self-governing through medical staff bylaws (Starr, 1982).

Maggie Mahar described the power shifting that has occurred among physicians and corporations. In her book, *Money-Driven Medicine*, Mahar points out that corporations are gaining power and control. Insurers routinely address physicians as "vendors" because that is how they are perceived within the corporate culture of insurance (2006, p. 340). Physicians are provided profit-and-loss reports that assess their productivity and metrics that evaluate the cost effectiveness of their work. Physicians are becoming alienated and angry because of the consistent emphasis on the financial bottom line. Some primary care physicians are opting for concierge practices that charge patients an up-front premium so that physicians can spend more time with them (Hartzband & Groopman, 2009).

The corporatizing of health care seems to be expanding beyond physicians to include nurses. Insurance giant UnitedHealth Group is targeting its nurses to teach them subjects such as economics and budget planning. It is no longer enough for nurses to simply concentrate on caring for their patients. Because the health care environment is becoming more business focused, nurses also need a better understanding of how their decisions affect health care costs. There are also plans to design business classes for the graduate-level nursing curriculum at the University of Minnesota (Newmarker, 2009).

But doctors do not have the same basis of power as large corporations, which is business confidence. The economy as well as the government's tax revenues depends on business confidence (Starr, 1982, p. 377). The relative importance of business confidence was demonstrated with the recent Congressional approved bailouts of the financial and automotive industries. Even though the majority of Americans opposed the bailouts and strongly voiced opposition, Congress overrode the will of the people to restore business confidence.

CONCLUSIONS

It may be that business is solving some of the problems that have confounded politicians and health policy makers for decades. For example, access to basic primary health services is problematic for too many Americans. Those who live in rural and other underserved areas often must travel to neighboring urban areas to see a primary care physician. The uninsured and underinsured forego needed care or end up seeking basic health services in an emergency department. But digital doctors' visits and Web consultations may ease access problems in a variety of ways, including reducing costs.

Grace Turner, the president of the Galen Institute, a research organization that focuses on health and tax policy, made the following observation in response to a story in the *Wall Street Journal* (May 14, 2007):

> Take note, Congress: The market is providing cheaper medicines, more affordable care—and it is also helping the uninsured. A Harris Interactive poll conducted in March (sic 2007) for the Wall Street Journal said that 22% of those visiting the clinics were uninsured. Wal-Mart says that half of its clinic visitors are uninsured. (Turner, 2007)

Business appears to be aggressively pursuing a variety of different strategies and ventures to help contain and hopefully reduce health care costs. From retail clinics to digital doctor's visits to on-site clinics, business is taking action. But even if business's efforts are successful, can the market ensure access to care? The shortage of primary care physicians, which is expected to worsen, will mean that many Americans will not have a regular source of care for primary health services.

Even those who live in health care hubs such as Boston, which is home to major medical centers, are having trouble gaining access to primary care. In Boston, the city's health department started a telephone referral service to connect its residents with primary care physicians who are accepting new patients. The city's mayor, Thomas M. Menino, organized a task force to figure out how to get more primary care doctors to work in the city. The mayor unsuccessfully objected to permitting retail clinics that are staffed by nurse practitioners to provide primary care services. The mayor has expressed a negative view of these clinics, including the fact that profiting off of sick people is wrong (Smith, 2008).

Although there is little evidence as yet that retail clinics are profitable, there is evidence that the uninsured are using retail clinics. Two major studies have informed us of this fact: one funded by the Rand Corporation (Mehrotra et al., 2008) and the other by the Robert Wood Johnson Foundation (Tu & Cohen, 2008). In addition, we have information that retailers are trying to help the uninsured. Walgreens has announced it will offer free clinic visits to the unemployed and uninsured for the rest of the year. Tests and routine treatment for minor ailments will be provided through Walgreens walk-in retail clinics (Yahoo News, 2009).

Will retail health care continue to drive costs down? Beyond that, will retailers lead the way to a more extensive array of affordable and convenient health care services? In the short term, the prices charged by retailers are considerably less expensive than those charged in traditional health care settings such as a physician's office or the emergency department. However, there is speculation that as insurers continue to increase their coverage of retail clinic visits, overall care costs could accelerate.

In a major study done by a larger insurer, HealthPartners in Minneapolis, Minnesota, researchers used claims data to examine 628,513 episodes of care that occurred during a four-year period. Researchers raised concerns because even though the cost of retail clinic visits are low, the costs are rising at about 3 percent per year.

Researchers further speculated that ultimately retail clinics might contribute to overall cost increases by inducing patients, who normally would use over-the-counter remedies, to instead visit a retail clinic because of affordability (Thygeson, Van Vorst, Maciosek, & Solberg, 2008).

Alternatively, because retail clinics offer a new access point for patients, fewer patients will delay seeking professional help and not enter the health care system much sicker, requiring more resources. Business would likely be satisfied with that outcome.

REFERENCES

Associated Press. (2007a, August 10). *Concerns rise over retail health clinics.* Retrieved August 13, 2007, from MSNBC.com: http://www.msnbc.msn.com/id/20215467/page/2/print/1/displaymode/1098/.

Associated Press. (2007b, December 6). *Waiting for flights offers time for flu shots.* Retrieved June 12, 2008, from Nytimes.com, *New York Times*: http://www.nytimes.com/2007/12/06/us/06flu.html?ei=5088&en=a5e5beda20bc2f55&ex=135.

Associated Press. (2009, April 22). *AMA plans one-stop electronic shopping for docs.* Retrieved April 22, 2009, from Yahoo News: http://search.yahoo.com/search;_ylt=A0oGkkzcAQhLrT0BN5Mqk6B4?p=AMA+plans+one-stop+electronic+shopping+for+docs&fr2=sb-top&fr=404_news&sao=0.

Balancia, D. (2007, December 12). *Disney Resort to build medical facility.* Retrieved December 12, 2007, from Florida Today: http://floridatoday.com/apps/pbcs.dll/article?aid=20071212/breankingnews/.

Barry, P. (2009, April). The new face of health care. *AARP Bulletin, 50*(3), 12–14.

Berry, L. L., Mirabito, A. M., & Berwick, D. M. (2004, Summer). A health care agenda for business. *MIT Sloan Management Review, 45*(40), 56–64.

Beckham, D. (2002, July/August). Emulating Wal-Mart. *Health Forum Journal, 45*(4), 37–38.

Booth, C. (2005, August 7). *Clinic saves money for county workers and government.* Retrieved August 7, 2005, from Tennessean.com: http://www.tennessean.com.

Broden, S. (2004, December 6). *New clinics offer quick treatment—County employees receive don't have to miss much.* Retrieved May 25, 2009, from *The Daily News Journal*: http://www.dnj.com.

Brownlee, S. (2007). *Overtreated: Why too much medicine is making us sicker and poorer.* New York: Bloomsbury.

Business Wire. (2008, October 29). *Health Net expands TRICARE access through RediClinics in Virginia.* Retrieved November 6, 2008, from CNBC.com: http://www.cnbc.com/id/27433731/site/14081545/.

Clark, K. (2005, October 17). The case for healthcare. *U.S. News & World Report, 139*(14), 36–38.

Claxton, G., et al. (2007, September/October). Health benefits in 2007: Premium increases fall to an eight-year low, while offer rates and enrollment remain stable. *Health Affairs, 26*(5), 1407–1416.

Collins, S. R., & Kriss, J. L. (2008). The public's views on health care reform in the 2008 presidential election. *The Commonwealth Fund.*

Colliver, V. (2008, December 21). *At more U.S. employers, the doctor is in.* Retrieved December 22, 2008, from SFGate.com: http://www.sfgate.com/cgi-bin/article.cgi?f=/c/a/2008/12/20/BUPR14LPC3.DTL.

Consumer Reports. (2009, April). When you need care fast. *Consumer Reports on Health, 21*(4), 6.

Crate, S., & Siefkin, K. (2005, December 12). *Whole health management to operate on-site wellness center at The Scotts Miracle-Gro Company.* Retrieved December 12, 2005, from Wholehealth.net: http://www.wholehealthnet.com/files/pdf/wh_pressrelease_scotts20051226.pdf#search=%22on-site%20health%20or%20wellness%20clinic%22.

Crounse, B. (2008). *Healthcare goes retail: In-and-out checkups.* Retrieved December 12, 2008, from Microsoft Health Care Providers, Microsoft Health Care Providers Official Site: http://www.microsoft.com/industry/healthcare/providers/businessvalue/housecalls/retailhealthcare.mspx.

Dossia. (2006, December 6). *Major U.S. employers join to provide lifelong personal health records for employees.* Retrieved May 26, 2008, from Dossia.org: http://www.dossia.org/news-events-media/media-center/doc_download/17-dossia-launches-.

Dossia. (2007, September 17). *Dossia gains momentum toward providing employees with personal, private, portable and secure health records.* Retrieved May 26, 2008, from Dossia.org: http://www.dossia.org/news-events-media/media-center/doc_download/12-dossia-gains-momentum.

Economist. (2006, December 7). *Wal-Mart and other big firms are pushing for electronic medical records.* Retrieved December 11, 2006, from Economist.com: http://www.economist.com/business/printerfriendly.cfm?story_id=8381456.

Felland, L. E., Hurley, R. E., & Kemper, N. M. (2008, May). Safety net hospital emergency departments: Creating safety valves for non-urgent care. *Center for Studying Health System Change, No. 120,* 1–4.

FierceHealthcare. (2007a, September 5). *Interview: Dr. Steve Cooley, CEO, SmartCare Family Medical Centers.* Retrieved July 24, 2008, from FierceHealthcare.com: http://www.fiercehealthcare.com/node/7934/print.

FierceHealthcare. (2007b, October 8). *Trend: Urgent care clinic industry expanding again.* Retrieved January 29, 2008, from FierceHealthcare: http://www.fiercehealthcare.com/node/8269/print.

Freddie Mac. (2004, September 21). *Freddie Mac opens free, on-site health center for employees.* Retrieved January 14, 2008, from Freddie Mac: http://www.freddiemac.com/news/archives/corporate/2004/wellness_092104.html?printpage=yes.

Freking, K. (2006, December 7). Electronic health records get boost. *Orlando Sentinel*, p. C3.

Freudenheim, M. (2007). *Company clinics cut health costs.* Retrieved January 14, 2007, from *New York Times*: http://www.nytimes.com/2007/01/14/business/14clinic.html.

Freudenheim, M. (2009, May 12). *Hospitals begin to move into supermarkets.* Retrieved May 12, 2009, from *The New York Times*: http://www.nytimes.com/2009/05/12/business/12clinic.html.

Garcia, J., Powers, S., & Clarke, S. K. (2008, April 21–27). CHD Meridian to run Disney Clinic. *Orlando Sentinel*, p. 8.

Giovis, J. (2008, February 7). *Blue Cross and Blue Shield opens store in Pembroke Pines.* Retrieved February 7, 2008, from South Florida Sun-Sentinel.com: http://www.sun-sentinel.com/business/sfl-flzinsureretail0207sbfeb07,0,602895,print.story.

Goldeen, J. (2008, June 6). *S.J. General to link patients, doctors via video.* Retrieved March 10, 2009, from Recordnet.com: http://www.recordnet.com/apps/pbcs.dll/article?aid=/20080606/a_news/806060338.

Goldstein, J. (2008). *Big insurers pay for online doctor visits.* Retrieved April 1, 2008, from *The Wall Street Journal*: http://blogs.wsj.com/health/2008/03/31/big-insurers-pay-for-online-doctor-visits/?mod=wsjblog.

Harris, S. (2008, September). *Open for Business: Health Systems Explore Retail Clinics.* Retrieved December 2, 2008, from Association of American Medical Colleges: http://www.aamc.org/newsroom/reporter/sept08/clinics.htm.

Hartzband, P., & Groopman, J. (2009, January 8). Money and the changing culture of medicine. *The New England Journal of Medicine, 360*(2), 101–103.

Healthcare News. (2006, November 8). *Toyota builds employee health clinic in new factory to reduce health care cost.* Retrieved January 14, 2008, from News-Medical.net: http://www.news-medical.net/print_article.asp?id=20920.

Herrick, D. (2006). *Consumer-Driven Health Care (CDHC) is leading to new models for the delivery of medical services.* Retrieved December 6, 2006, from Consumer Driven Health Care: http://healthcare.ncpa.org/commentaries/consumer-driven-health-care-cdhc-is-leading-to-new-models-for-the-delivery-of-medical-services.

Hoover, J. N. (2006, December 11). *Companies unveil data pool to assault health care costs*. Retrieved December 11, 2006, from TechWeb—The Business Technology Network: http://www.techweb.com/article/printablearticlesrc.jhtml?articleid+196602778.

Hospital Impact. (2006, July 19). *Retail clinics—Coming to a drug store near you?* Retrieved January 24, 2008, from Hospitalimpact.org: http://www.hospitalimpact.org/index.php/scoop/2006/07/19/retail_clinics_coming_to_a_drug_store_ne.

Howard, M. R. (2007, November 1). *Healthy*. Retrieved February 5, 2008, from Florida Trend: http://www.floridatren.com/print_article.asp?aid=47806.

Hunt, K. G. (2007, November 15). *NBGH supports retail health clinics*. Retrieved May 25, 2008, from Business Insurance Daily: http://www.businessinsurance.com/article/20071115/news/200011615.

Immediate Care Business. (2009). *Cleveland Clinic teams with Minute-Clinic*. Retrieved February 21, 2009, from Immediate Care Business Official Site: http://www.immediatecarebusiness.com/hotnews/cleveland-clinic–minuteclinic-team-up.html#.

Jones, S. M. (2009, March 28). *Drug prices: Wal-Mart/Caterpillar plan may drive down employer health-care costs*. Retrieved May 9, 2009, from Chicagotribune.com: http://archives.chicagotribune.com/2009/mar/28/business/chi-sat-wal-mart-pharmacy-mar28.

Kaiser Family Foundation. (2006, November 8). *Toyota builds employee health clinic in new factory to reduce health care costs*. Retrieved January 14, 2008, from News-Medical.Net, The Medical News: http://www.news-medical.net/news/2006/11/08/20920.aspx.

Kennedy, K. (2008, February 4). *Disney World, Publix among those planning to open on-site clinics*. Retrieved February 5, 2008, from The Ledger.com, Polk County Business Journal: http://www.theledger.com/apps/pbcs.dll/article?aid=/20080204/news/802040308/1178.

Klepper, B. (2008, March 28). *What worksite and retail clinics mean for the primary care crises*. Retrieved October 2, 2008, from Health Care Policy and Marketplace Review: http://healthpolicyandmarket.blogspot.com/2008/03/what-worksite-and-retail-clinics-mean.html.

LaPenna, A. M. (2009, March/April). Workplace medical clinic: The employer-redesigned "company doctor." *Journal of Healthcare Management, 54*(2), 87–91.

Lawton, C. (2009, March 5). *Cough, cough. Is there a doctor in the mouse?* Retrieved March 10, 2009, from WSJ.com, *The Wall Street Journal*: http://online.wsj.com/article/sb123621447433335269.html?mod=-article-outset-box.

Lohr, S. (2009, March 11). Wal-Mart plans to market digital health records system. *The New York Times*, p. B1.

Mahar, M. (2006). *Money-Driven Medicine*. New York: Harper Collins Publishers.

Maurer, H. (Ed.) (2006, October 9). A $4 Rx. *The Business Week*, 34.

Mehrotra, A., Wang, M. C., Lave, J. R., Adams, J. L., & McGlynn, E. A. (2008, September/October). Retail clinics, primary care physicians, and emergency departments: A comparison of patients' visits. *Health Affairs*, 27(5), 1272–1282.

Merchant Medicine. (2008, November 11). *On-site employer-sponsored clinics*. Retrieved November 11, 2008, from Merchant Medicine: http://www.merchantmedicine.com/consultingservices.cfm.

Merchant Medicine. (April 2, 2009a). *On-site employer clinics—Disruptive innovation times two*. Retrieved April 7, 2009, from Merchant Medicine: http://www.merchantmedicine.com/news.cfm?view=33.

Merchant Medicine. (April 2, 2009b). *Retail clinics: 2008 year-end review and 2009 outlook, many closures in 2008 but the market continues to expand*. Retrieved April 7, 2009, from Merchant Medicine: http://www.merchantmedicine.com/news.cfm?view=21.

Merrill, M. (2009, April 13). *Minnesotans to receive access to a virtual clinic*. Retrieved April 13, 2009, from Healthcare IT News, Physician Practices & Ambulatory Care: http://www.healthcareitnews.com/news/minnesotans-receive-access-virtual-clinic.

Newmarker, C. (2009, February 27). *UNH to teach business to nurses*. Retrieved March 17, 2009, from Minneapolis/St. Paul Business Journal: http://twincities.bizjournals.com/twincities/stores/2009/03/02/story4.html.

Perin, M. (2008, August 1). *Retail Health Clinics Reopen with New Model*. Retrieved February 3, 2009, from Houston Business Journal: http://houston.bizjournals.com/houston/stories/2008/08/04/story4.html?t=printable.

Perrone, M. (2009, March 11). *Wal-Mart to enter electronic medical records arena*. Retrieved March 11, 2009, from Yahoo Official Site, Yahoo News: http://search.yahoo.com/search?p=walmart+to+enter+electronic+medical+records&fr=ush-news&ygmasrchbtn=Web+Search.

Pierce, O. (2007). *Survey: Workers want healthcare from jobs*. Retrieved January 2, 2008, from UPI Health Business: http://www.upi.com.

Plott, B. (2007, October 29). *The doctor is in . . . In Fairchild City Hall*. Retrieved October 30, 2007, from Al.com, The Birmingham News: http://www.al.com/printer/printer.ssf?/base/news/11936459052 76220.xml&coll=2.

Powers, S. (2008, October 15). *Disney opens health care center for employees*. Retrieved October 16, 2008, from OrlandoSentinel.com, Orlando Sentinel: http://blogs.orlandosentinel.com/business_tourism _aviation/2008/10/disney-opens-he.html.

Revolution Health Group. (2005, October 5). *Revolution Health Group announces initial acquisitions; Key executives tapped to build comprehensive consumer-driven health company*. Retrieved January 2, 2006, from Internet News Unlimited: http://www.ip97.com/revolution

_health_group_announces_initial_acquisitions_key_executives
_tapped_to_build_comprehensive_consumer_driven_health_bbch
.aspx.

Robeznieks, A. (2007, November 11). Look who's buying retail. *Modern Healthcare, 37*(46), 26–28.

Rosen Hotel. (2008). *Rosen Hotel & Resorts employee benefits*. Retrieved February 5, 2008, from Rosenhotels.com: http://www.rosenhotels .com/benefits.asp.

Smith, S. (2008). *City adds a doctor referral service*. Retrieved August 1, 2008, from Boston.com: http://www.boston.com/news/local/ articles/2008/08/01/city_adds_a_doctor_referral_service/.

Solantic. (2008a). *Flu shot guarantee*. Retrieved November 10, 2008, from Solantic.com: http://www.solantic.com/flu.asp.

Solantic. (2008b, July 25). *Solantic urgent care issues health debit cards*. Retrieved November 10, 2008, from Immediate Care Business: http://www.immediatecarebusiness.com/hotnews/health-debit-cards.html.

Starr, P. (1982). *The social transformation of American medicine*. New York: Basic Books.

Strupp, D. (2007, July 30). *Private equity firm's $100M to fund Solantic's growth plans*. Retrieved November 10, 2008, from Jasonville Business Journal: http://www.bizjournals.com/jacksonville/stories/ 2007/07/30/daily1.html.

Thygeson, M., Van Vorst, K. A., Maciosek , M. V., & Solberg, L. (2008). Use and costs of care in retail clinics versus traditional care sites. *Health Affairs, 27*(5), 1283–1292.

Traugot, C. L. (2007, October 5). *Urgent clinics, pharmacies adding outlets for walk-ins*. Retrieved January 29, 2008, from Triangle Business Journal: http://triangle.bizjournals.com/triangle/stories/2007/10/08/ focus3.html.

Tu, H. T., & Cohen, G. R. (2008). Checking up on retail-based health clinics: Is the boom ending? *The Commonwealth Fund, 48*, 1–12.

Turner, G. (2007, May 14). Customer health care. *The Wall Street Journal, The Wall Street Journal Online*, A17.

Welch, D. (2008, July 29). *Health-care reform, corporate-style*. Retrieved December 22, 2008, from BusinessWeek: http://www.business week.com/print/magazine/content/08_32/b4095000246100.htm.

Wells, S. J. (2006, May 28). The doctor is in-house. *HR Magazine, 51*(4).

Wertheimer, L. K. (2008). *Firms give health advise for a price*. Retrieved June 23, 2008, from Boston.com: http://www.boston.com/news/health/ articles/2008/06/23/firms_give_health_advice_for_a_price?mode.

Wessel, H. (2008, January 15). Ocoee to join growing list of employers opening clinics. *Orlando Sentinel*, pp. C1–C2.

Wikipedia. (2008). *Richard Lynn Scott*. Retrieved November 10, 2008, from Wikipedia: http://en.wikipedia.org/wiki/Richard_Lynn_Scott.

Wohl, J., & Zimmerman, D. (2009, January 14). *Walgreen offers health program for businesses.* Retrieved January 14, 2009, from Reuters.com: http://www.reuters.com/article/idustre50d4vj20090114.

Wojcik, J. (2007, December 10). *Employers spot link between health, profit.* Retrieved January 16, 2008, from Business Insurance: http://www.businessinsurance.com/article/20071209/issue01/100023612.

World Research Group. (2008). *On-site employee health clinic summit.* Retrieved May 29, 2009, from World Research Group: http://www.worldrg.com/showconference.cfm?confcode=hw10023&field=whoattends.

Wyden, R., & Bennett, B. (2008, May/June). Finally, fixing health care: What's different now? *Health Affairs, 27*(3), 689–692.

Yahoo News. (2009, March 31). *Walgreens giving free care to jobless and uninsured.* Retrieved April 22, 2009, from Yahoo News: http://search.yahoo.com/search;_ylt=A0geu_ULIghLzt4AKwVXNyoA?p=walgreens+giving+free+care+to+jobless+and&fr2=sb-top&fr=ush-news&sao=0.

Yang, C. (2005, April 11). Another case entirely. *Business Week,* 64–68.

Yu, R. (2008). *Health care businesses take off at airports.* Retrieved April 8, 2008, from USA Today: http://www.usatoday.com/travel/flights/2008-04-07-airport-clinics-pharmacies_n.htm.

Zieger, A. (2009, March 9). *Patient teleconsults become more common.* Retrieved March 10, 2009, from Fierce Health IT: http://www.fiercehealthit.com/node/8300/print.

zz_Ferris, N. (2008, June 18). *4 Percent of U.S. doctors use EHRs, new study finds.* Retrieved March 31, 2009, from Government Health It: http://govhealthit.com/articles/2008/06/4-percent-of-US-doctors-use-EHRs-new-study-finds.

zz_Ferris, N. (2008, November 12). *Survey: Hospital EHR adoption rate is below 12 percent.* Retrieved March 31, 2009, from Government Health It: http://govhealthit.com/articles/2008/11/survey-hospital-ehr-adoption-rate-is-below-12-percent.

Chapter 9

The Globalization of Health Care

The assumption that "all health care is local" is pervasive in the industry. However, there have been periods when that assumption has been challenged. For example, in the 1970s and 1980s, for-profit as well as nonprofit hospitals attempted to build hospital chains. The idea behind this type of expansion was that the hospital's brand would attract new patients. Hospitals ultimately failed in these efforts because it turned out that a national or regional brand was less important to consumers than the reputation of the local hospital and the connection with the community it served.

In 2009, national retailers are trying to build markets for their in-store retail clinics by collaborating and subsequently co-branding with local hospitals and health systems. Walmart, in particular, seems to be focusing on a co-branding strategy with local health care organizations. More than 50 in-store Walmart retail clinics are owned and operated by local hospitals and health systems (Jenks, 2009).

However, the notion that "all health care is local" may be less relevant for the future. Just as American manufacturing has engaged in outsourcing to cut expenses, consumers, employers, and insurers are looking beyond the United States to discover opportunities to reduce health care costs. During the next few years, it is expected that the world will probably see more investment, medical staff, and patients crossing borders in order to achieve increased access to affordable care (Economist, 2008).

Globalization is not new to health care. For some time now, American hospitals have outsourced their record keeping, transcription of doctors' notes, and X-ray analysis (*Economist*, 2008). However, developments in technology have facilitated global interactions and remote management of clinical and administrative operations. Consequently, more and more health care is going global.

Another factor influencing the trend is the upgraded quality of care offered abroad. Many of the physicians in countries such as India have trained in the United States and returned to establish high levels of quality and performance at their hospitals. Furthermore, quality is waning as an issue because hospitals outside of the United States are increasingly obtaining accreditation by the respected Joint Commission International, a nonprofit organization that evaluates quality and safety and is an affiliate of the main accrediting body for U.S. hospitals (McQueen, 2008; *Economist*, 2008).

In addition, many of the hospitals and facilities outside of the United States have been built from scratch or modernized and upgraded to attract patients from all over the world. Finally, health care in overseas facilities costs significantly less than it does in the United States (*Economist*, 2008). Medical care in countries such as India, Thailand, and Singapore can cost as little as 10 percent of the cost of comparable care in the United States. For example, the cost of heart-bypass surgery in India is $10,000 compared with $130,000 in the United States (Richman, Udayakumar, Mitchell, & Schulman, 2008).

This chapter seeks to answer the following questions:

1. Does America face a competitive threat from global health care organizations?
2. What is medical tourism, and how is it expected to change the delivery of health care both in the United States and throughout the world?
3. Is there a "global" role for retail health clinics?
4. Why are prestigious U.S. academic health centers such as the Cleveland Clinic and Johns Hopkins forming global partnerships with hospitals and health facilities throughout the world?
5. What lessons can be learned from other countries?

MEDICAL TOURISM

Medical tourism involves patients traveling, usually a great distance, to obtain medical care. Medical tourism can be "domestic" and involve travel several hours away to a nearby state. It can also involve travel halfway around the world. Medical tourism is not a one-way street. It can be both outbound and inbound. Outbound travel refers to patients who travel outside the United States for care. Inbound characterizes patients from other countries who travel to American facilities for treatment (Keckley & Underwood, 2008).

For example, British patients have traveled to the Mayo Clinic and other facilities in the United States for decades. They have done so because of delays in surgeries and diagnostic procedures under their government health plan (Economist, 2008). In 2008, more than 400,000 non-U.S. residents were expected to seek care in the United States and spend almost $5 billion for their health services. These patients represent about 2 percent of all users of hospital services in the United States. Most of the patients come from the Middle East, South America, and Canada (Keckley & Underwood, 2008, p. 19).

Americans also travel to foreign countries for non-FDA approved treatments. Actor Steve McQueen made headlines when he went to Mexico in the 1970s to take an experimental treatment for lung cancer. In 2009, a former Charlie's Angel, Farrah Fawcett, revealed that she obtained an alternative treatment for her cancer in a German facility.

The concept of medical tourism is not new. The term, however, is new. It evokes an image of the patient as a "medical tourist," one who goes sightseeing either before or after a serious hospital procedure (Grassi, 2006; Konrad, 2009). It has been defined in a variety of ways, but is generally believed to encompass the following:

> Medical tourism refers to the act of traveling to another country to seek specialized or economical medical care, well being and recuperation of acceptable quality with the help of a support system. (Keckley & Underwood, 2008, p. 6)

The world market for medical tourism is predicted to be about $60 billion and to grow to $100 billion by 2010, although estimates vary. Over 35 countries are serving approximately one million medical tourists annually. There are at least ten regions that are considered to be *hot spots* for medical tourism:

1. Hungary
2. Gulf States

3. Mexico

4. Costa Rica

5. Brazil

6. South Africa

7. Malaysia

8. India

9. Thailand

10. Singapore (Keckley & Underwood, 2008)

Until recently, few Americans traveled abroad for medical care other than elective cosmetic and dental surgeries. But that is rapidly changing. Medical tourism is increasingly viewed as a growing trend among U.S. health care consumers (McQueen, 2008). The Deloitte Center for Health Solutions, a consulting group, has estimated that 750,000 Americans traveled abroad for medical care in 2007. This number is expected to increase to 6 million by 2010 (Keckley & Underwood, 2008).

An April 2009 the Gallup Poll reported that many Americans, especially the uninsured, are willing to travel outside of the United States for medical procedures if quality of care is comparable and costs are lower (Commins, 2009). Deloitte's 2008 Survey of Health Care Consumers revealed that nearly 40 percent of consumers would go overseas for medical care if the cost was reduced by half and quality was comparable to that of U.S. facilities. The Deloitte survey revealed gender differences as men were much more likely than women to consider a trip abroad for treatment, by a margin of 44.5 percent to 33.3 percent (Deloitte, 2008a).

Americans with insurance are beginning to see some atypical options in their network of providers: facilities and physicians that are located outside of the United States. Some employers and insurers are beginning to cover treatment overseas for major surgical procedures, including heart surgeries and hip and knee replacements. And they are making travel abroad more attractive by offering incentives, including bonuses and reimbursement of travel costs (McQueen, 2008).

Large U.S. insurers are also starting to put international medical tourism programs in place. WellPoint, the nation's largest health insurer, is conducting a pilot program with Serigraph Inc., a specialty graphics company with operations in Wisconsin, Mexico, and Asia. The program offers U.S. employees the option to travel to India to have surgery on a nonemergency basis (Healey, 2009).

Blue Cross Blue Shield of South Carolina created a subsidiary for medical tourism called Companion Global Healthcare. The company maintains a network of international doctors and hospitals, including Bumrungrad International Hospital in Bangkok, the Parkway Group Healthcare in Singapore, and hospitals in Turkey, Ireland, and Costa Rica (McQueen, 2008; Einhorn, 2008).

Shopping Around for Health Care

The majority of candidates for medical tourism are uninsured and underinsured people who are paying out of pocket and are looking for health care bargains (Konrad, 2009). *Shopping around for health care is possible because of the Internet and the growth of medical tourism companies that assist patients in finding affordable alternatives to traditional providers. What motivates patients is not only the high cost of care in the United States, but also the lack of transparency.

For example, an electrician with nine children was told in 2008 that he needed triple bypass surgery, which would cost $80,000 *or more* (Starke, 2009). By using the Internet, the electrician found a facility that would do the surgery for $13,200, The Galichia Heart Hospital in Wichita, Kansas. Galichia participates in a domestic medical tourism program run by Healthbase Online, a Boston-based company that locates U.S. hospitals offering specialty surgeries at lower prices than traditional providers. Healthbase also runs an international medical tourism program (Starke, 2009).

When an uninsured 56-year-old male car salesman from Yakima, Washington, was told that he needed a new hip, the 56-year-old went on the Internet and searched the phrase "free hip replacement." Even though he did not get the surgery for free, the cost was only $15,000, or one quarter of what was quoted by the local hospital. The car salesman received his new hip at the Gleneagles Medical Centre Penang, Malaysia. To locate this international alternative, the car salesman used a company that he found on the Internet, an Illinois-based medical tourism agency called Med-Retreat (Van Dusen, 2007).

From Niche to Mainstream? Or Out of Business?

Medical tourism is a *niche* business: a small market segment of the overall health care industry. Will medical tourism become *mainstream*? There is little evidence to suggest what the future holds for medical tourism. Despite growth projections, there are many factors that could inhibit the growth of medical tourism, especially when it involves travel abroad. If either employers or insurers do not find the quality outcomes or costs comparable to what could be obtained in the United States, they will cease covering treatment at foreign facilities. The uninsured might also be deterred from seeking care abroad if government policies restrict travel. This could be either for political reasons such as unrest or violence or it could be purely for health reasons. For example, if there were an outbreak or quarantine in a country, travel would become impossible.

U.S.-based organizations have emerged to facilitate care overseas for patients as well as to perform a clearinghouse function for companies wishing to outsource their employees' health care. Examples of these organizations include MedSolution, GlobalChoice Healthcare, IndUShealth, Planet Health Care, and MedRetreat (Grassi, 2006; Van Dusen, 2007). Even though many of these organizations act as patient representatives for finding treatment abroad, often providing assistance with travel arrangements, patients still are at increased risk if anything goes wrong during the procedure.

According to a 2008 report on medical tourism by Deloitte, a consulting group, medical tourism programs are successfully positioned to attract international patients. Many of the earlier drawbacks, especially for developing countries, such as communications, transportation, water, sewer, and power, have been overcome by strong economic development programs (Keckley & Underwood, 2008).

Some opposition for medical tourism has come from U.S. doctors. The American Medical Association (AMA) has suggested the need for oversight and medical tourism guidelines. The American Academy of Orthopaedic Surgeons has raised concerns for patient safety, especially blood transfusions and possible contamination with viral pathogens such as HIV or hepatitis C (MQueen, 2008).

Labor unions have also opposed efforts to establish medical tourism programs. For example, in 2006, the United Steelworkers stopped a patient who was scheduled to fly to India for a procedure (McQueen, 2008). With the economic downturn, especially for the automotive industry, it will be interesting to see how unions deal with the prospect of medical tourism in the future.

Meanwhile, there will likely continue to be a global market for health care as long as there are patients from other countries who can pay higher costs than the country's residents. For example, Apollo Hospitals, India's largest hospital and health system, proactively works to attract patients from the United States (Healey, 2009).

HOSPITALS AND HEALTH SYSTEMS

America's hospitals and health systems are also looking overseas to establish new markets and sources of revenues. Experts estimate that each foreign venture can be expected to yield hundreds of thousands of dollars in revenue for the institution (Van Dusen, 2008). Examples of prominent U.S. academic health centers that are involved in some of the international collaborations include the following:

1. Cleveland Clinic
2. Cornell Medical School
3. Duke Medical School
4. Partners Harvard Medical International
5. Johns Hopkins International
6. Memorial Sloan Kettering
7. University of Pittsburgh Medical Center
8. Columbia University Medical School (Keckley & Underwood, 2008)

The trend of large, reputable American hospitals going international is fairly recent. Some believe that the trend was at least in part the result of the aftermath of September 11, 2001, when it became difficult for travelers, including medical tourists, from the Middle East and other regions to obtain U.S. visas. Prior to September 11, these patients represented a healthy revenue stream for American hospitals because they paid in cash or the government took care of the bills. Hospitals that did not want to lose this revenue began to go overseas to provide the care (Van Dusen, 2008).

In addition, the growth of a middle class in Asia and the Middle East has expanded the market for more sophisticated health care services. However, many of the countries do not have the facilities or staff to respond to the increased demand. American hospitals, especially those affiliated with a medical school, can help these countries by providing specialists, training, and facilities management.

What do the American hospitals get in return? Foreign revenue, which has become especially attractive in light of the economic downturn and tight budgets for hospitals and universities. Revenue from international projects can be used to fund teaching, research, and construction projects back in the states (Fitzpatrick, 2008; Van Dusen, 2008). Below are examples of three prestigious academic health centers that have global partnerships.

Cleveland Clinic

The Cleveland Clinic is proactive in its approach to international collaborations and has aggressively pursued relationships abroad. It already has established campuses in Toronto, Canada, developed an affiliation with the International Medical Center in Jeddah, Saudia Arabia, and is partnering with the government of the United Arab Emirates to construct a 360-bed, multispecialty Cleveland Clinic Abu Dhabi hospital (Van Dusen, 2008). The Clinic is also exploring new contracts in China, Guatemala, Brazil, Egypt, and India (Fitzpatrick, 2008).

The University of Pittsburgh Medical Center

The University of Pittsburgh Medical Center is the largest health system and largest employer in southwestern Pennsylvania. Because the Medical Center's revenues are down, it has pursued a variety of international relationships. The Medical Center operates private hospitals in Ireland and also manages two Irish cancer centers. It also operates facilities and programs in the United Kingdom, the Mediterranean, and the Middle East. For example, in Qatar, the Medical Center provides consulting services and physicians for a medical system. Meanwhile, in Italy, it manages a transplant center in Palermo (Fitzpatrick, 2008).

The Medical Center claims that it has been well rewarded for its global initiatives, citing profitable operations and sizable management fees in the millions of dollars. For example, in Qatar, the Medical Center is being paid $100 million over a five-year period to train physicians and provide expertise to four hospitals. However, its international and commercial division is the smallest of the Medical Center's three business lines. Furthermore, in the first six months of its 2008 fiscal year, the division lost $4 million compared with $52 million in profit generated by its insurance initiative (Fitzpatrick, 2008).

Johns Hopkins

Not all American universities and hospitals are aggressive in their approach to international collaboration. Johns Hopkins has been more conservative. The institution is focusing on medical projects that involve academic and clinic advisement rather than building new facilities. Johns Hopkins has ties with Japan, India, Canada, Turkey, Singapore, China, Chile, and Panama. Johns Hopkins also has a long-term affiliation with the United Arab Emirates, including the management of a 400-bed hospital in Abu Dhabi (Keckley & Underwood, 2008; Van Dusen, 2008).

Much of what academic health centers can accomplish overseas reflects the improvements in technology. For example, the University of Pittsburgh Medical Center uses telecommunications systems to link the two Irish cancer centers that it operates, one in Waterford and the other in Dublin, to its Hillman Cancer Center back home in Pittsburgh (Fitzpatrick, 2008).

RETAIL CLINICS IN THE UNITED KINGDOM

The United Kingdom has a national health service (NHS) sponsored by the government, which affords residents universal coverage. Despite universal coverage, patients have access problems and have difficulty seeing their doctors during working hours. One solution being attempted to resolve some of these problems is the United Kingdom's version of the retail clinic.

In 2008, J. Sainsbury, one of Britain's largest supermarket chains, became the first in the country to offer a visit to the family doctor in one of its stores. Through a program called *Doctors InStore*, patients will have access to basic primary care services after working hours and on weekends. In this way, the British can combine shopping with doctor's appointments, which is pretty much what many Americans are already doing with retail clinics (Werdigier, 2008).

What was truly remarkable about this venture was that a team of government-financed doctors will see patients. This is unlike retail clinics in the United States, where the clinics are private enterprises (Werdigier, 2008). Meanwhile, J. Sainsbury's competitor, a supermarket chain called Asda, is reportedly signing a similar agreement that will permit family doctors to operate clinics at two of its stores (Times Online, 2008).

Doctors InStore is the brainchild of Mohammed Jiva, a 35-year-old family doctor in the Manchester area of England. Doctors InStore was founded in 2007 to foster a joint venture between

NHS and the stores (Primed Services, 2008). In the United Kingdom, there is a shortage of primary care physicians, which creates access problems for patients. There are 1,600 patients for each family practitioner. This contrasts with 325 patients for every doctor in the United States. Dr. Jiva observed a growing demand from patients to book appointments in the evening or on weekends and conceptualized the in-store clinic as a way to satisfy patients' needs for convenience (Werdigier, 2008).

The NHS offers free medical consultations, provided Britons see doctors from their home area. Thus if they work at a distance from home, seeing a doctor means returning to their home area. It has been estimated that employees cost the British economy approximately $2 billion of work time spent traveling to their home areas for a doctor's appointment (Werdigier, 2008).

The British government is supportive of using in-store clinics to expand access to care and solicited bids from stores to participate in a pilot program. The clinics operate on two evenings a week and also on Saturdays (BBC News, 2008). In addition, the doctors use their own laptops to access patient records and make referrals or update records (Times Online, 2008). The funding for the pilot program as well as two other trials originates from taxpayers' money. Doctors are expected to initially see only up to 70 patients per week (Times Online, 2008).

The British experiment with in-store clinics has similarities and differences compared with retail clinics in the United States. American retail clinics represent free enterprise and are owned by the private sector. In the United Kingdom, the clinics are a hybrid collaboration of public and private sectors. The goals for American clinics are similar to those of the United Kingdom: convenience and expanded access to basic primary care services. The financial goals are shared, too. The British government wants the clinics to succeed because they will save the British economy roughly $2 billion dollars annually for "unproductive" time that employees spend seeking medical care. The stores that partner with the British government want the clinics to succeed because they hope to piggyback on their success with increased foot traffic. In the United States, retail clinics are aimed at enhancing productivity and profitability, too.

CONCLUSIONS

Global health efforts can be expected to continue, especially if health care costs continue to increase. However, there is little evidence concerning the impact of these efforts to be able to determine if globalization is a plus or a negative for the U.S. health care system. For example, even though medical tourism appears to reduce health care costs for employers, insurers, and patients, it also potentially negatively affects physicians, hospitals, and other providers in the U.S. health care system.

Deloitte Center for Health Solutions has developed figures showing the impact of medical tourism on the U.S. health care system. Specifically, medical tourism represents $15.9 billion in lost revenue for U.S. health care providers. Given projections for growth of medical tourism, from 750,000 in 2007 to 15.75 million in 2017, the potential loss of revenue for U.S. providers in year 2017 is a staggering: $228.5 to $599.5 billion (Keckley & Underwood, 2008, p. 14).

How will the United States respond to competition overseas? If Indian hospitals have American trained doctors that can perform open heart surgery for $6,000 compared to $100,000 in the United States, why would insurance companies insist that patients stay in America for their care, especially if the quality is certified as comparable?

Unlike the United States, India's environment is seen to be more conducive to innovation because of its competitive and more open marketplace. In India, hospitals are permitted to commercialize technologies as offshoots of the health care delivery business. For example, they spin off companies that manufacture medical equipment and thus keep the prices low. Or they reengineer service delivery models to maximize use of capital equipment. An example of this is doing outpatient radiology studies by day and doing inpatient studies overnight. In this way, periods of down time for expensive equipment are minimized (Richman et al., 2008).

However, there are opportunities for American businesses and for health care providers to develop global partnerships. For example, China's health care system needs a complete overhaul. Its public hospitals have been criticized for their lack of access, huge fees, and poor services. The lack of a functioning health care system is a source of widespread unhappiness among the Chinese public. In addition, remote villages and less developed cities are in need of improvements in service delivery and access (Yahoo News Malaysia, 2009).

American academic medical centers could collaborate with the Chinese in improving its health care system. Retailers could partner with the Chinese, too. For example, Walmart, which already has stores in China, could offer retail clinics as an additional portal of entry. Retail clinics would enhance access for the Chinese who lived in proximity to Walmart stores. In addition, Walmart might consider adopting telemedicine clinics for in-store clinics. The telemedicine clinics could address problems of those living in remote areas.

Furthermore, U.S. hospitals and health systems might find it advantageous to co-brand with Walmart for overseas ventures much the same way they have co-branded American clinic offerings. Walmart already has a few retail clinics in its Walmart stores in Mexico. The clinics are owned by Samoho, a Mexico City–based company that has also opened clinics in three Miami-area pharmacies whose customers are mostly Spanish speaking (Goldstein, 2008).

REFERENCES

BBC News. (2008, March 3). *Supermarket starts store GP pilot*. Retrieved March 5, 2008, from BBC News: http://news.bbc.co.uk/1/hi/england/manchester/7274453.stm.

Commins, J. (2009, May 30). *Poll: Sizeable minority of Americans would consider medical tourism*. Retrieved May 20, 2009, from HealthLeaders Media: http://www.healthleadersmedia.com/content/233354/topic/ws_hlm2_gbl/poll-sizeable-minority-of-americans-would-consider-medical-tourism.html.

Deloitte. (2008a). *2008 Survey of health care consumers*. Retrieved May 28, 2009, from Deloitte: http://www.lindsayresnick.com/resource_links/consumers_health_care_2008.pdf.

Deloitte. (2008b). *Medical tourism: Emerging phenomenon in health care industry*. Retrieved May 26, 2009, from Deloitte: http://www.deloitte.com/dtt/article/0,1002,cid%253d225733,00.html.

Doctors InStore. (2007). *Doctors InStore—About us*. Retrieved March 5, 2008, from Doctors InStore: http://www.doctorsinstore.co.uk/about.html.

Economist. (2008, August 14). *Operating profit*. Retrieved January 20, 2009, from The Economist: http://www.economist.com/opinion/displaystory.cfm?story_id=11919622.

Einhorn, B. (2008, March 24). Outsourcing the patients. *Business Week*, 36.

Fitzpatrick, D. (2008, February 26). *UPMC to manage hospital in Ireland as continuation of expansion strategy*. Retrieved February 27, 2008, from Pittsburgh Post-Gazette: http://www.post-gazette.com/pg/08057/860408-28.stm.

Goldstein, J. (2008, August 15). *How do you say "retail clinic" in Spanish?* Retrieved August 18, 2008, from *The Wall Street Journal*: http://

blogs.wsj.com/health/2008/08/15/how-do-you-say-retail-clinic-in-spanish/.

Grassi, D. M. (2006, November 15). *Offshoring U.S. patients no cure for ailing healthcare system*. Retrieved April 28, 2009, from RenewAmerica: http://www.renewamerica.us/columns/grassi/061115.

Hawkes, S. (2008, February 22). *Feeling unwell? Just pop down to the supermarket to see the GP*. Retrieved March 5, 2008, from Times Online: http://business.timesonline.co.uk/tol/business/industry_sectors/retailing/article3412598.ece.

Healey , J. (2009). *Health care tourism, now covered by insurance?* Retrieved April 28, 2009, from Los Angeles Times: http://opinion.latimes.com/opinionla/2009/04/health-care-tourism-now-covered-by-insurance.html.

Jenks, S. (2009). In a hurry? Clinics offer speedy care. Retrieved November 24, 2009, from http://www.floridatoday.com/article/20091117/NEWS01/911170320/In-a-hurry?=Clinics-offer-speedy-care.

Keckley, P. H., & Underwood, H. R. (2008). *Medical tourism—Consumers in search of value*. Retrieved May 28, 2008, from Deloitte: http://www.deloitte.com/dtt/cda/doc/content/us_chs_medicaltourismstudy(1).pdf.

Konrad, W. (2009). *Going abroad to find affordable health care*. Retrieved March 25, 2009, from *New York Times*: http://www.nytimes.com/2009/03/21/health/21patient.html.

McQueen, M. P. (2008, September 30). *Paying workers to go abroad for health care*. Retrieved September 30, 2008, from *The Wall Street Journal*: http://online.wsj.com/article/sb122273570173688551.html.

Primed Services. (2008). *Doctors InStore*. Retrieved March 5, 2008, from PriMed Services: http://www.primedservices.co.uk/doctorsinstore.html.

Richman, B. D., Udayakumar, K., Mitchell, W., & Schulman, K. A. (2008, September/October). Lessons from India in organizational innovation: A tale of two heart hospitals. *Health Affairs, 27*(5), 1260–1270.

Sarasoh-kahn, J. (2008, July 28). *Wal-Mart enters telemedicine*. Retrieved August 1, 2008, from Health Populi: http://www.healthpopuli.com/2008/07/wal-mart-enters-telemedicine.html.

Starke, A. B. (2009, April). Affordable surgery closer to home. *AARP Bulletin*, 10.

Times Online. (2008, March 4). *Sainsbury doctors set up shop*. Retrieved March 5, 2008, from Times Online: http://www.timesonline.co.uk/tol/life_and_style/health/article3478919.ece.

Van Dusen, A. (2007, May 29). *Outsourcing your health*. Retrieved January 27, 2009, from Forbes: http://www.forbes.com/2007/05/21/outsourcing-medical-tourism-biz-cx_avd_0529medtourism.html.

Van Dusen, A. (2008, August 8). *America's top hospitals go global*. Retrieved January 27, 2009, from Forbes: http://www.forbes.com/2008/08/25/american-hospitals-expand-forbeslife-cx_avd_0825health.html.

Werdigier, J. (2008, March 3). *Combining grocery shopping with doctors' appointments*. Retrieved March 5, 2008, from *The New York Times*: http://www.nytimes.com/2008/03/03/business/worldbusiness/03docs.html?_=3&oref=slogin&pagewanted.

Yahoo News Malaysia. (2009, January 22). *China to spend $124 billion on medical reforms*. Retrieved January 22, 2009, from Yahoo News Malaysia: http://search.yahoo.com/search?p=china+to+spend+%24124+billion+on+medical+reforms&fr=ush-news&ygmasrchbtn=Web+Search&pvid=H6o7E0geui_qmpzMSwac.QDjGO4T00sIIy MADcCR.

Chapter 10

Future Predictions and Implications of Retail Clinics for All Stakeholders

In this chapter we will consider the future development of retail health clinics and the implications of this future for all stakeholders. At this point in time there are both actual and potential facilitators of retail clinic development as well as actual and potential impediments to such development. The relative strength of these facilitators and impediments will vary from time to time and place to place.

For example, it is possible that facilitators will be stronger than impediments in the short term, but impediments will be stronger longer term. This scenario would imply that retail clinics would grow rapidly in the short run, but slow down in growth longer term. It is also possible that they will grow rapidly in some parts of the country (i.e., the South and the Midwest) while growing slowly in the Northeast and West Coast due to more extensive legislative and regulatory barriers.

A recent report by the Deloitte Center for Health Solutions discusses two growth waves for retail clinics and predicts their future growth based on this analysis. The first phase of wave one, which occurred from 2006 to 2008, was growth driven by acquisitions. The second phase of wave one, from 2008 to 2012, is a focus on profitability and development of a foundation for the next phase. Wave two, from 2012 to 2014, is growth driven by new markets and services (Keckley et al., 2009).

Merchant Medicine, a leading tracker of retail clinic operators, has suggested that the market may top out at 4,000 in 2015 (Merchant Medicine, 2009). The 65 percent annual growth rate of clinics from 2000 to 2007 will likely slow to 15 percent from 2008 to 2009. Then the growth rate will likely remain between 10 and 15 percent from 2010 to 2012. Finally, Deloitte expects the growth rate in clinics to accelerate above 30 percent from 2013 to 2014 (Keckley et al., 2009).

It is also important to point out that the future will be very much impacted by what retailers, retail clinic providers, physicians, hospital and health systems, and other stakeholders choose to do in response to the recent growth of retail clinics. For example, if the major providers and other stakeholders choose to partner with retail clinics, the growth prospects could be very bright. If they choose to not collaborate, but compete, retail clinics could still grow, although more slowly. If they choose to compete politically through opposition in Congress and state legislatures, retail clinics may grow very slowly. In fact, all of the major stakeholders have reflected a wide variety of positions that vary to some degree from stakeholder to stakeholder and from place to place.

Facilitators include problems with the current primary care system, recent changes in health insurance, expanding insurance coverage of retail clinics, customer satisfaction with such clinics, current Joint Commission on the Accreditation of Healthcare Organizations (JCAHO) accreditation to validate quality, electronic communications by such clinics, high levels of customer satisfaction, and potential health care reform to insure the uninsured. Impediments include potential increased legislation and regulation to stifle the growth of retail clinics as well as actual and potential increased market competition.

We will also examine the implications of retail clinics and strategies health care providers might adopt to address the challenges of managing and responding to such clinics. In this chapter we will look at strategies that could be adopted by retailers, retail clinic providers, physicians, and hospitals/health systems. Finally, we will look at the implications of retail clinics and strategies other stakeholders might adopt to respond to them. Among these other stakeholders are patients/consumers, insurers, employers, and public officials/policy makers.

The authors will conclude with some scenarios for the future of retail clinics. These scenarios as well as other materials in this chapter draw heavily on the work of Mr. Kenneth Peach, president of Future Vision Group of Orlando in his presentation at the Third Annual Retail Health Clinic Summit (Peach, 2009).

FACILITATORS TO FUTURE RETAIL CLINIC GROWTH AND DEVELOPMENT

Table 10.1 examines actual and potential facilitators and impediments to future retail clinic growth and development. The first facilitator is the fact that many consumers have difficulty arranging timely appointments at convenient hours with their primary care physician. This problem is expected to worsen in the years ahead as a result of an increasing shortage of primary care physicians. A second facilitator is the fact that health insurance coverage is beginning to cover retail clinics, which increases incentives for insured patients to use them. In some cases, the expanded insurance coverage also incorporates incentives for enrollees to use them in preference to other primary care alternatives such as physician practices, urgent care clinics, and emergency departments.

Traditional health insurance has also seen major increases in coinsurance and deductibles in recent years, which has meant that the insured are paying a higher percentage of their health costs out of pocket. For basic health services, these consumers could minimize their out-of-pocket costs if they use retail clinics. The growth of medical savings accounts also gives the consumer greater control and more incentive to choose lower cost options, such as retail clinics.

Not all states currently have retail clinics available for their citizens. Either the retailers themselves have not yet felt that these markets can support retail clinics or they would like to open retail clinics in these states but face significant regulatory barriers. Nevertheless, retail clinics continue to grow and have become more available to more citizens over the past two or three years. It is likely they will continue to grow in the future, at rates that will be determined by the relative strength of the facilitators and impediments outlined in Table 10.1.

As retail clinics have grown and become more available, they have become more familiar to and more accepted by consumers. Therefore, retail clinic growth and enhanced availability has itself become a facilitator for future growth.

TABLE 10.1   Actual and Potential Facilitators and Impediments to Retail Clinic Growth and Development

Actual and Potential Facilitators	Actual and Potential Impediments
(1) Problems in achieving timely appointments and convenient hours with physicians	
(2) Expanding insurance coverage for retail clinics	(1) Potential increased federal, state, and local legislation and regulation of retail clinics: • AMA Resolution 705 • Possible malpractice cases • Union pressure for shorter work shifts • State laws governing which clinical professionals may perform which functions • State mandated regulation of retail clinic staffing ratios • Necessity for government approval of new technology • Higher insurance requirements for retail clinics • Potential conflicts of interest related to retail clinics
(3) Increases in medical savings accounts, insurance deductibles, and coinsurance	(2) Actual and potential increased market competition: • Online services offered by other providers • Lab and diagnostic services in retail settings • More customer-friendly physician practices • An increased emphasis on "medical homes" • Focused clinical management programs • Site based and mobile imaging services • Increased online and telephonic services • E-commerce • Traditional providers opening their own retail clinics

(4) Growth and enhanced availability of retail clinics around the country	
(5) Customer satisfaction with retail clinics	
(6) Current JCAHO accreditation of retail clinics	
(7) E-Care	
(8) Potential health care reform to insure uninsured population subgroups	

Customer satisfaction in retail clinics is quite high as noted in previous chapters. This is due to convenience, geographic accessibility, and low prices. Such consumer satisfaction should facilitate future clinic growth.

Since one concern raised by critics is potential lower quality of services at retail clinics, the fact that some clinics (i.e., Minute-Clinic) have already achieved JCAHO accreditation and others are seeking such accreditation serves as a positive indicator of quality. In turn, such quality indicators should serve to facilitate retail clinic growth in the future. Recent research found that patients received higher quality care for routine conditions in retail clinics compared with physician offices, urgent care centers, and emergency departments (Mehrotra, 2009).

Retail health clinics already use electronic medical records, which allows them to transmit patient records to physicians, insurers, and other providers. As a result, retail clinics have an advantage in the area of E-Care. For example, e-prescriptions allow the provider to have the prescription ready when the patient checks out, and it also reduces medical errors. As a result, the patient receives higher quality care in a more efficient manner. This situation should also facilitate the growth of retail clinics.

Currently, health care reform initiatives are ongoing with the goal of targeting uninsured or underinsured population subgroups including low-income, minorities, and others. As a result, we expect that these newly insured subgroups may increase demand for retail clinic services in the future.

IMPEDIMENTS TO FUTURE RETAIL CLINIC GROWTH AND DEVELOPMENT

The first major impediment to future retail clinic growth and development is the possible increased federal, state, and local legislation and regulation of retail clinics. AMA Resolution 705 was passed by the AMA House of Delegates at its June 2007 meeting in Chicago. This resolution attacked the safety and quality of retail clinics and called for legislative initiatives to examine their potentially negative impact on consumers. As the AMA and other physician groups lobby their state legislatures, there is a potential for negative legislation and regulation, which will impede the growth of retail clinics or may possibly exclude them entirely from some states. Although none has occurred thus far, there is also the possibility of a large malpractice case that could create a negative image of retail clinics in the minds of consumers and stimulate possible negative legislation and regulation at the state level.

Labor unions may also pressure state legislatures to regulate hours of work, work shifts, and appropriate functions and staffing ratios for physician assistants and nurse practitioners practicing in retail clinics. Higher insurance requirements for retail clinics and lack of approval for necessary clinic technology could be other impediments to clinic growth. Finally, it is possible that a court may find clinics that sell pharmaceuticals while also providing retail clinic services might be guilty of a conflict of interest even if they do not require patients to fill prescriptions in their own pharmacy.

The second major actual or potential impediment for clinics would be increased market competition from other providers. These other providers include physician practices, hospitals, and health systems as well as employers who choose to offer clinics for their own employees. Any or all of these competitors might offer online services, lab and diagnostic services, more customer-friendly practices, focused clinical management practices, global services of various types, and e-commerce. They may also open their own retail clinics in direct competition to current retailers and retail clinics.

IMPLICATIONS AND STRATEGIES OF RETAIL CLINICS FOR HEALTH CARE PROVIDERS

In this section we will address the implications of current trends in retail clinics for the following four health care providers:

retailers, retail clinic providers, physicians, and hospitals/health systems (see Table 10.2). For all of these providers we recommend defining the patients as the primary customers.

Retailers

Retailers should market their clinics in terms of product, price, place, and promotion. This means they should make consumers aware of the nature of their product (i.e., what they provide and what they do not provide), the relatively low price compared to other primary care alternatives, the geographic place or places this service is available, and where consumers can find additional information. Although retail clinics currently provide very basic primary care services, they may want to also gradually expand their offerings beyond basic services to chronic care, patient education, diagnostics, and portable clinic imaging. In so doing, they should assess the financial feasibility of these services for particular markets.

Retailers may also want to partner with a variety of delivery organizations including retail clinic providers, physician groups, and hospital and health systems. They may also consider co-branding their clinics with well-known partners such as Cleveland Clinic and Mayo Clinic. They should also invest directly in lobbying their state legislatures and Congress to fight legislation and regulation to restrict their activities. They might also consider collaborating with employers to provide on-site health services directly to employees.

Retail Clinic Providers

To combat criticism from physicians, retail clinics have established evidence-based clinical protocols. It is also important that they utilize telemedicine to access high-quality partners and seek or maintain JCAHO accreditation. Again, the clinics themselves should market their services based on products, prices, place, and promotion as already mentioned for retailers.

Clinic providers should continue to expand their electronic medical records since this gives them a competitive advantage relative to some physician practices that do not yet have electronic medical records. They should also comply with all medical protocols for the particular services they provide. Their retail mind-sets should focus on selling small quantities of services directly to the

TABLE 10.2   Retail Clinic and Health Care Provider Implications and Strategies

Retailers:

- Define the patients as the primary customers
- Market clinics in terms of product, price, place, and promotion
- Gradually expand clinic offerings beyond basic services (i.e., chronic care, patient education, diagnostics, portable clinic imaging)
- Partner with a variety of delivery organizations including physician groups, hospital and health systems, and retail clinic providers
- Co-brand clinics with well-known partners such as Cleveland Clinic and Mayo Clinic
- Assess financial feasibility for particular clinic services in particular markets
- Lobby state legislatures and Congress to avoid restrictive legislation and regulation.
- Collaborate with employers to provide on-site health services directly to employers

Retail Clinic Providers:

- Define the patient as the primary customer
- Establish evidence-based clinical protocols
- Utilize telemedicine to access high-quality partners
- Seek and maintain JCAHO accreditation
- Market services based on products, prices, place, and promotion
- Establish and expand electronic medical records
- Comply with medical protocols
- Think retail by selling small quantities of services directly to the consumer
- Continually modify hours of operation and schedules to respond to patient needs
- Partner with retailers, medical groups, and hospitals/health systems

Physicians:

- Define the patient as your primary customer
- Monitor retail clinics to emulate their successful innovations
- Avoid overscheduling of patient visits to allow sufficient time for communication
- Invest in technology that serves your patients (i.e., email, silent pagers, etc.)
- Modify hours of operation and scheduling to respond to patient needs
- Communicate with patients online and through telephonic services
- Partner with retailers and retail clinics through written contracts providing mutual referrals
- Expand concierge medicine offerings to bring services to the patient
- Compete in the market rather than in the legislature
- Avoid criticizing retail clinics based on unproven allegations of low quality.

Hospitals/Health Systems:

- Define the patient as your primary customer
- Partner with retail clinics through written contracts providing mutual referrals
- Provide basic care for basic needs
- Look for ways to use resources more efficiently, such as utilization of nurse practitioners and physician assistants
- Consider differentiating your services by opting out of basic care and competing on the basis of clinical and service quality
- Utilize telemedicine to co-brand with well-known partners
- Invest in technology that serves your patients (i.e., email and silent pagers)
- Standardize services through computerized clinical protocols
- Monitor retail clinics and emulate their successful innovations
- Experiment with different models of service delivery such as back clinics provided in retail settings
- Move some advanced lab and diagnostic services to retail settings
- Utilize e-commerce to market some diagnoses, prescriptions, and "do-it-yourself" treatment supplies online
- Communicate with patients and provide patient education online and through telephonic services
- Offer on-site clinics for various employers
- Enhance customer service through easier appointment scheduling, reduced waiting times, and seamless service

consumer. Their clinic model should be flexible so that they modify hours of operation and schedules to respond to patient needs. Finally, they should be prepared to partner with and develop mutual referrals to retailers, medical groups, and hospitals/health systems.

Physicians

Physicians should monitor health clinics to emulate their successful innovations that meet patient needs. Based on previous research, we know that patients criticize overscheduling of patient visits, which does not allow sufficient time for communication. Obviously, physicians have a trade-off here since they are under pressure from insurers to see more patients in a given time period.

Physicians also need to invest in technology that serves their patients, such as email and silent pagers. They may also want to modify their hours of operation and appointment system to respond to patient needs. For example, leaving time for some patients without appointments each day may enhance patient satisfaction. They may also want to communicate with patients online and through telephonic services without requiring patients to come to the office for all communications.

Physicians should also be open to partnering with retailers and retail clinics through written contracts providing mutual referrals. They may also want to initiate or expand concierge medicine offerings to bring services directly to the patient. Finally, they may want to choose to compete in the market, rather than in the legislature, and avoid criticizing retail clinics based on unproven allegations of low quality.

Hospitals/Health Systems

Hospitals and health systems may want to consider partnering with retail clinics through written contracts providing mutual referrals. They may also want to look for ways to use their resources more efficiently such as utilization of nurse practitioners and physician assistants to provide services not requiring physicians.

They may also consider whether they want to provide basic care for basic needs or simply opt out of basic care and compete on the basis of clinical and service quality. For example, they could use telemedicine to co-brand with well-known partners, thus enhancing their image of clinical quality. They could also invest in technology that serves their patients such as email and silent pagers.

Similar to retail clinics, they may want to standardize their basic services through the use of computerized clinical protocols. They may also want to monitor retail clinics to emulate their successful innovations. Health systems may also want to experiment with different models of service delivery such as back clinics, advanced lab and diagnostic services, provided in retail settings.

These systems could also utilize e-commerce to market some diagnoses, prescriptions, and "do-it-yourself" treatment supplies online. They could also communicate with patients online and through telephonic services. They could also offer on-site clinics for various employers. Finally, they could enhance customer service through easier appointment scheduling, reduced waiting times, and seamless service.

RETAIL CLINIC IMPLICATIONS AND STRATEGIES FOR OTHER STAKEHOLDERS

Table 10.3 outlines implications and strategies of the growth of retail clinics for other (nonprovider) stakeholders. These include patients/consumers, insurers, employers, and public officials/ policy makers.

Patients/Consumers

Patients and consumers need to seek out and support retail clinics for their basic health services if such clinics are available in their community. They also need to pressure employers and insurers to insure such services and monitor retail clinics to assess potential new offerings. Finally, they should become more proactive in seeking out lower cost convenient alternatives to traditional primary care services by using technology.

Insurers

Insurers should include retail clinics in all of their insurance products. They should also provide financial incentives for their enrollees to use these clinics in preference to other primary care alternatives. Finally, they may want to consider opening their own primary care retail clinics.

Employers

Employers should include retail clinics in their employee insurance products. They should also make sure these products create

TABLE 10.3   Retail Clinic Implications and Strategies for Other Stakeholders

Patients/Consumers:	Insurers:
• Seek out retail clinics for basic health services if available in your community • Pressure employers and insurers to insure retail clinic services if available in the community • Monitor retail clinics to assess potential new offerings • Become proactive in seeking out lower cost, convenient alternatives to primary care services by using technology.	• Include retail clinics in insurance plans • Provide financial incentives for enrollees to use retail clinics in preference to urgent care centers, primary care physician practices, and hospital emergency departments for relevant, basic services • Consider opening insurer-owned primary care retail clinics
Employers:	Public Officials/Policy Makers:
• Include retail clinics in employee insurance products • Create incentives for employees to utilize retail clinics in preference to other primary care alternatives • Consider opening your own on-site health clinic or outsourcing these services to a retail clinic provider such as Walgreens's Take Care Health • Local governments may consider contracting with retail clinic providers for basic health services for their employees	• Enhance educational opportunities for nurse practitioners and physician assistants to ensure adequate supply for retail clinics • Refrain from legislative and regulatory initiatives to stifle the growth of retail clinics • Stop playing politics with health care • Consider allowing veterans to receive services outside the VA system in retail clinics

incentives for employees to use retail clinics in preference to other, more expensive primary care alternatives. They should also consider opening their own on-site health clinic or outsourcing these services to a retail clinic provider. Local government employers may consider contracting with retail clinic providers for basic employee health services on-site.

Public Officials/Policy Makers

Since retail clinics draw heavily upon the employment of nurse practitioners and physician assistants in staffing their clinics, an adequate supply of each is necessary for continued retail clinic growth. Policy makers should ensure that institutions of higher education produce a sufficient quantity and quality of both so that this staffing model may be continued in the future.

Public officials may also need to refrain from legislative and regulatory initiatives to stifle the growth of retail clinics. Federal policy makers may also want to consider allowing veterans to receive health services outside the VA system in retail clinics.

THREE POSSIBLE FUTURE SCENARIOS

The influence of retailers on health care leads to three possible future scenarios for the U.S. health care system. The first scenario, *retail by default*, involves a future in which the government has become distracted by world events and continuing economic problems. In this future, the retail movement has managed to make its health care ventures profitable and consumers are satisfied with convenience, affordability, and quality. The second scenario, *government intervention*, reflects a future in which the health care system is reformed by government fiat. The Democrats have enough votes to champion a national health plan and do so. The third scenario, *more of the same*, promises a continuation of the status quo in which health care costs continue to escalate and powerful institutional forces inhibit disruptive innovations.

Retail by Default

Under the retail by default scenario retailers end up changing the health care system because the government fails to do so. The government is distracted by world events and continuing economic problems and subsequently fails to enact a national health plan. Meanwhile retailers have continued to move into health care markets and experiment with new models of care delivery. In particular, retail clinics have begun to offer chronic and preventive care services. Retailers quickly adopt technology and disruptive innovations to expand their capacity to reduce prices and enhance convenience for consumers.

Retailers also move into health markets overseas, offering a variety of health care services through their international stores. Emergency department overcrowding is reduced because hospitals can direct patients to retail clinics and other alternative sites for basic health services. Employer on-site clinics persist and manage to reduce the cost of health benefits. Medicare and Medicaid programs provide incentives to their enrollees to use retail clinics and online alternatives for basic care needs. The Department of Veterans Affairs also has granted access to its enrolled veterans to use low cost retail clinics rather than to travel to Veterans Affairs facilities. This is very helpful in reducing travel time and cost to veterans, especially those living in areas that are at a distance from Veterans Affairs facilities.

Government by Intervention

In the government by intervention scenario, the Democrat Congress passes a plan to nationalize health insurance. Because any outlines for a national health plan are ill-defined at this point, it is difficulty to speculate on what will occur. However, given the government's experience with intervening in banking and automotive industries, it is highly likely that whatever plan they choose to implement will mean significant upheaval for the health care system.

For example, everyone will have access to insurance. However, because there is a shortage of primary physicians and because there are shortages of health professionals in rural and underserved areas, it is likely that universal insurance coverage will create more access problems. In order to control costs, it is also possible that some type of rationing system will be implemented. Finally, taxes will be increased to cover the government health plan because the financial bailouts of other industries have occupied a disproportionate of future government spending.

More of the Same

Under the more of the same scenario, the future will probably not be much different from the health care system that is in place currently. Under this scenario, retailers abandon U.S. health care markets because increased regulation and competition interfered with profitability. Instead, retailers take their health care innovations overseas and generate profits. The government will "tinker" with programs to reduce costs, but never realize control over them. Powerful institutional forces will persist in impeding any attempts at national health reform. Taxes will increase to cover the escalating health care costs, especially for Medicare and Medicaid programs.

Under this scenario, costs will continue to increase. Insurers and employers will apply utilization controls and disincentives in the form of higher premiums and co-payments. Consumers will find themselves paying more for health care and spending even more time waiting to see the doctor.

The Most Probable Future

We believe that elements of all three scenarios are likely in the future. That is, we may have some elements of "retail by default" as whatever health care reform passes does not directly interfere with the growth of retail clinics. So clinics will continue on their current growth trajectory with some additional financial support as some previously uninsured subgroups become insured and some of that support benefits retail clinics. However, scenario two (government intervention) is also likely as Congress passes new health reform legislation and some form of rationing is implemented. Such rationing could involve a willingness to pay for certain services at certain predetermined levels. This might create incentives for patients to receive more of their services in retail clinics.

It is also likely that in the future we will see both increased regulation and increased competition for retail clinics. This could mean their growth rate may slow as regulation impedes their growth in some places and competition impedes their growth in some places.

CONCLUSIONS

Only retailers could have affected the significant changes we have seen in health care in the past decade. They have implemented the disruptive innovation known as the retail clinic. They have used electronic technology to maximize efficiency, convenience, and affordability. They have also used nurse practitioners and physician assistants to achieve the same goals. They have taken health care out of the doctor's office.

The impact of retailers is very significant. They have created lower costs for all participants, increased access to primary care, and are a possible remedy to the primary care physician shortage. For these reasons, the retail revolution can be categorized as a major disruptive innovation. Retail clinics are not a fad. They are a trend driven by consumers who seek more value. They are continuously evolving as they take on new forms that are responsive to local market pressures. They are also responsive to the concerns of employers and insurers for lowering health care costs. These retail clinics are providing basic health care services with a high level of satisfaction.

We are beginning to experience an increase in collaboration between retailers and traditional health care providers such as hospitals and health systems. Neither envisioned such collaboration initially. Both assumed that they would remain independent and grow their own services without collaboration with the other. However, retailers and hospitals/health systems have united for their mutual self-interest in terms of co-branding and foot traffic. Obviously, the retailers gain credibility by partnering with well-known, local providers, and these providers gain foot traffic from the retailers, which can also enhance referrals to their facilities. So it is a "win-win" strategy for both.

These partnerships should not be viewed as marriages between the two parties. Both are experimenting with attempts to achieve mutual self-interest. What they are really involved in is a committed relationship. This relationship will continue as long as both parties benefit from it. If the time comes when either or both parties fail to achieve their financial goals, then the relationship will dissolve.

Retail clinics have managed to reach a previously underserved population: the uninsured and the underinsured. With technology such as telemedicine retail clinics have the potential to expand into rural communities and beyond the United States into global communities. If the growth of retail clinics falters, underserved groups already facing access pressures may suffer from the potential loss of alternative sources of primary care (i.e., retail clinics) more than the rest of the population (Tu & Cohen, 2008).

Retail clinics have evolved at a time when our health care system was floundering and not meeting the needs of a significant portion of the population. They filled a need in the niche market of basic primary care services. They did so with an emphasis on quality, convenience, and consumer choice. At this point, they have the potential to "move upstream" to more sophisticated services such as chronic and preventive care. They have established high standards of quality, employ competent clinicians, and use electronic medical records and ongoing quality improvement mechanisms. Among the most important of these is evidence-based clinical practice.

While retail clinics have obviously filled a niche at the present time and have the potential to expand beyond that niche, we do not know at this time whether they will play a major or a minor role in our evolving future health care system. Retail clinics do provide a model of low cost, high quality, convenient, and cost effective care, which should be incorporated into our future health care system.

REFERENCES

Keckley, P. H., Underwood, H. R., and Gandhi, M. (2009). *Retail clinics: Update and implications.* Deloitte Center for Health Solutions.

Mehrotra, A. (2009). Retail medical clinics offer quality care. *Annals of Internal Medicine, 151,* 321–328.

Merchant Medicine. (2009). Retrieved November 24, 2009, from http://merchantmedicine.com/news.cfm/view=24.

Peach, K. (2009, May 29). *Sustaining success: Techniques for continuing and growing your retail health clinic business by partnering with the primary care market.* Third Annual Retail Health Clinic Summit. Orlando, FL.

Tu, H. T., & Cohen, G. R. (2008, December). Checking up on retail based health clinics: Is the boom ending? *The Commonwealth Fund. Issues Brief No. 1199.* New York: The Commonwealth Fund.

Index

About the Authors

MYRON D. FOTTLER is Professor and Executive Director of Programs in Health Services Administration at the University of Central Florida. Dr. Fottler has written many books on health care, most recently *Human Resources in Health Care* and *Achieving Service Excellence: Strategies for Health Care*. He has an MBA from Boston University and a Ph.D. in Business from Columbia University.

DONNA M. MALVEY is Associate Professor in Health Services Administration at the University of Central Florida. Dr. Malvey's research has addressed the needs of the changing health care environment as well as implications of these changes for health services administration education. She has a MHSA from The George Washington University and a Ph.D. in Administration-Health Services from the University of Alabama at Birmingham.

DATE DUE

JUN 0 1 2012			
GAYLORD			PRINTED IN U.S.A.